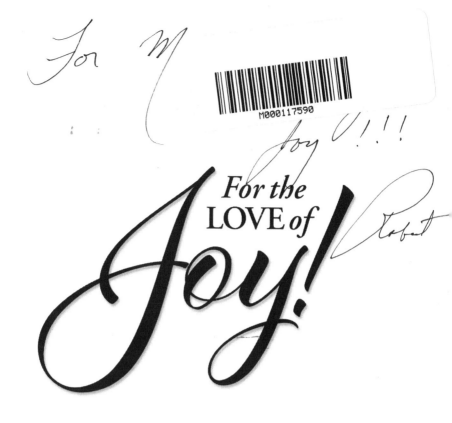

# For the LOVE of Joy!

## A 30-Day Adventure for Creating Joy in Your Life

*Because You Deserve More Joy,*
*More Love, More Health,*
*More Abundance And More Life!*

ROBERT MAX SCHOENFELD

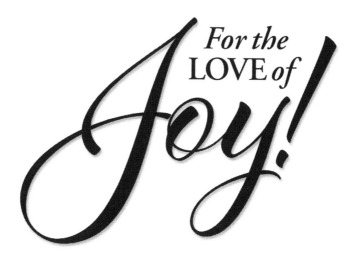

*For the*
LOVE *of*

# Living Your Magnificence!

Feeling how it feels to live
your Love, Joy, Beauty, Power,
Kindness, Integrity, Creativity,
Nobility and Magnificence.

Moving from Stress, Overwhelm, Depression,
Anger, Fear, Rage, Pain and Lack, to Love and Joy!

Dancing, Singing, Laughing, Eating and Loving
Your Way to More Joy, More Health, More Life!

*Be Still and Listen,*
*For Joy is Calling You,*
*Joy is Waiting for You,*
*For Where There is Joy There is Love,*
*And Where There is Love There is Peace.*
*For When You are In Peace the Splendor*
*Of Life Will Be Awakened In You!*
*So Be Joy, Be Love, Be Peace...*
*I Will Meet You There.*

# For The Love Of Joy

*A 30-Day Adventure for Creating Joy in Your Life*

Because You Deserve More Joy, More Love, More Health,
More Abundance, More Life

By Robert Max Schoenfeld

Cover and Interior Design by: Robert Lanphear
www.LanphearDesign.com

Guide and Journal Publications
Seattle, WA 98118


www.ExpandingJoy.org
Info@ExpandingJoy.org

ISBN  978-0-9744504-7-6  Soft Cover


Printed in the United States of America

This book is dedicated to everyone who has the
Inner Strength, Perseverance and Grace
to move from fear into Love.

A special thank you to the following world-inspiring and
inspirational leaders for their enlightened wisdom:
Panache Desai, Jo Dunning, Matt Kahn, Marie Manuchehri,
Jim Self, Neale Donald Walsch, Rikka Zimmerman
and to
Janee Pennington Watson and Abby Lodmer
for helping to make this book possible.

# Take a Selfie!

On the first day of *For the Love of Joy!*

Today's Date _____
Your First-Day Picture Here

At the finish of *For the Love of Joy!*

Today's Date _____
Your Picture Here

# Contents

# FOREWORD

## *I Am a Holder of The Dream*

Some years ago I was listening to a talk given by a nationally known author and speaker. She went on and on about how all of her close women friends have beautiful families – yet they are all taking medication for anxiety and depression.

When I heard this, it saddened me. I started to think to myself that there must be a better way.

Throughout my life I have been the holder of the dream that life can be a loving, joyful, abundant, peaceful, healthy and exciting adventure.

What if there is a way for us to stand in our magnificence and by doing so reduce the sadness, pain and lack in our lives while increasing – in some subtle yet powerful way – the love, joy, peace and abundance in our lives, in our families and in all life on earth?

This is my dream. I invite you to join me. For the next thirty days – and for the rest of your life thereafter – STAND IN YOUR MAGNIFICENCE, and watch as your life moves from pain and lack to love and abundance.

> *You may say that I'm a dreamer–but I'm not the only one…*
> —John Lennon

Let us dream together and create lives full of love, joy, beauty, creativity, generosity, gratitude, forgiveness, personal power, purpose, courage, nobility, romance and fun, leading to a brighter world for us, our families and for future generations.

In-Joy!

*Robert Max Schoenfeld*

# Introduction

What if life is designed to be Joyful and Loveful (Full of Love)? What if you are a Magnificent Being who has the wisdom and power to live in that full Magnificence? If over the next 30 days you wholeheartedly apply the exercises in this book, you will move more fully into your Magnificence, Joy and Love.

The goal in working through *For The Love Of Joy!* is to bring more love and light into your life and in so doing, have the darkness and mud (anger, shame, depression, guilt and sadness) fall away.

## What Is Your Wish For Your Life?

What would it feel like to be on a warm, private beach in Hawaii being held and touched romantically by your loving partner? How would it feel to be in the Swiss Alps having a glass of wine, telling stories and laughing with close friends? How would it feel to be clapping for your grandchild as she plays the lead in her school's performance of *Gone with the Wind*? What would it feel like to start your morning feeling refreshed, excited and ready to shine your Magnificence? How would it feel to fall into bed at the end of the day, feeling good about yourself, fulfilled and with a sense of well-being? What would it feel like to fully Love and Cherish yourself, to be Loved and Cherished by others, and to be fully Loved and Cherished by Life? Take a few moments and feel into these feelings. These are the joys of life and you are entitled to them. They are your birthright. If you desire something, it can be yours, but you must want it – really want it. Only then will you take the actions necessary to move from depression to joy, from fear to love, from lack to abundance.

You are about to go on a 30-day adventure that will move you towards living life with more zest, embracing a positive self-image, envisioning a brilliant future and feeling an overall sense of JOY!

There are no guarantees in life, but if you commit to the 30 actions in this book, your life will change for the better.

This is your life! Take charge – dig deeper into yourself than you ever have before, and make the commitment! Make it NOW!

## Make Today a Turning Point

This is not a book to help you deal with your anger, manage your rage, or battle your depression. This book will guide and inspire you to receive more JOY, BEAUTY and LOVE in your life – for where there is Joy, anger cannot exist; where there is Beauty, rage is released; and where there is pure Love, depression melts away like ice in the hot sun.

This is a 30-day adventure, so jump into it and have fun! The goal is for you – at the conclusion of this journey – to experience your life with more Love, Joy and Abundance.

From this time forward, your 24/7 mantra is: "*I Love You.*" Send *I Love Yous* to yourself and to every experience life brings your way— the good, the bad, and the . . .

Be kind to yourself, even if you miss a day, a few days, or even a week. We all slip up from time to time along the journey towards a better life. This adventure in Joy is all about moving you forward with Grace.

## Choose Life!

There is an old Jewish saying: "One who saves a single life is considered as if he saved an entire world." Today, commit to saving your life, thus saving the world.

Be the Tortoise along this path—Strong, Determined, Confident and Calm—and not the Hare—speedy, flaky, erratic and lazy. Take your time with this process, and make it fun. This is your Life, not a sprint to the finish line! There is a lot of helpful information in these pages, all of which is designed to help you move into a more joyous and love-filled life. Take it one day at a time and do not take on more than you can easily incorporate into your daily routine. As you move through your day, keep the vision of your goal in mind and enjoy being the Tortoise!

## The Power Of Love–The Power Of Self-Love

What if Love is all there is? What if all of life is just vibration? What if feelings of anger, sadness and pain are forms of Love vibrating at a very low level? What if Love, Joy, Beauty, Wisdom, Creativity, Connection, Peace, Enlightenment and Freedom are all forms of Love vibrating at a very high level? (See the Vibration of Love Chart on page 31). What if by raising your level of Self-Love all lower vibrations such as hate, anger, sadness, resentment, rage, jealousy, lack and pain will fall away? What if the true way to Joy, Success, Love and Fulfillment in your life will naturally manifest when you reach higher levels of Self-Love?

This book offers you many tools and exercises that are designed to directly and effectively raise your level of Self-Love.

To live in Love, Happiness and Joy is a choice. So choose Life! It takes commitment, courage and vision… and some heavy lifting… but you can do it! The rewards – a happier, more fulfilling and purpose-filled life – will make your effort worthwhile!

For the next 30 days, put yourself first and act like you are saving a life, because YOU *ARE* SAVING *YOUR* LIFE.

## Magnificence

You are a magnificent being who was uniquely made, by the Creator of the Universe, to shine your magnificence.

It is much easier to shine your magnificence when you are out of the mud (depression, anger, guilt, rage, shame, lack) and basking in the light and joy of living your true magnificence. Each day, as you move through this book, you will gain skills and insights that will bring more light and joy into your walk through life. Feel into the following question: What would it be like to live in my Magnificence?

## The Power Of Living Words

What if you have the power to transform your life through the words you think and speak? What if – by consciously choosing words that are joyful, healthy and positive – your experiences in life will become more joyful, healthier and positive?

Infuse your entire Being (emotional, physical and mental), with the essence of: I Am Courageous, I Am Loving, I Am Certain, I Am Capable, I am Gracious, I Am Forgiven, I Am Forgiving, I Am Beautiful, I Am at Peace and any other Power Words of your choosing. As you walk through your day, breathe these words into your Being, feel the essence of each word fill you with power, joy and peace – and watch your life change for the better!

This process of affirmation is not just a mental process; it is a much deeper experience, where every cell in your body—your entire essence—is enlivened with the feeling of Being Courage, Being Loving, Being Certain, Being Capable, Being Graciousness, Being Forgiven, Being Forgiving, Being Beauty and Being Peace.

You will learn how to go deeper into the power of Living Words on Day 6.

## Being In The Question

"Being in the question" is a wonderful way for the Universe to grant your every wish. What if the Universe loved you so much that your every command stimulated it to move heaven and earth to open the doors to fulfill your command beyond your wildest dreams? Feeling into the question (not looking for the answer) is trusting and allowing the Universe to bring you the Love, Joy, Health and Abundance you desire, in Divine timing.

**Being in the question – Take a moment to feel into:**

- ❖ What would it feel like to truly Love Myself?
- ❖ What would it feel like to truly Love My Life?
- ❖ What would it feel like to have a healthy body?
- ❖ What would it feel like to be financially abundant?
- ❖ What does it feel like to be confident?
- ❖ What does it feel like to be capable?
- ❖ What does it feel like to be neutral?
- ❖ What does it feel like to be happy?

Feel the joy of *being in the question* and allow the Universe to make it so!

Feel confident that the Universe is arranging life to make it happen – in its own timeline.

# Rumi

Rumi (1207–1273) was one of the greatest poets of all time. Rumi's poetry and philosophy sings truth and beauty to the heart, grace to life and light to the soul. His words help to open the heart to Joy and Knowing.

As you read his poems in this book, gently breathe the words into your heart and allow them to float in your Being.

# Join The Love Revolution

The Love Revolution is happening all over the world. This is your personal invitation to join in on the fun. To be a member of the Love Revolution, the only requirement is to send Love to yourself and to all that life brings you. Join today, and watch your life sing with Love, Joy and Beauty.

## Your Mission

Your mission – should you accept it – is to bring more Love, Joy and Beauty into your life for the next 30 days (and for the rest of your life), everything else comes second!

## Sweetness

Look for ways to put some sweetness in your life every morning, afternoon and evening.

A fun way to add sweetness is to apply the essential oil of rose or sweet orange to your face and neck as a perfume or cologne. The scent of rose and sweet orange will put a smile on your face and warm your heart.

**Being in the question, ask yourself:** "What new Sweetness would I like to experience today?"

*Find the sweetness in your own heart.*
*That you may find the sweetness in every Heart.*
—**Rumi**

## Smile

What if a simple smile has the power to raise your level of joy and feeling of well-being? Research proves that smiling helps to produce endorphins and oxytocin that create feelings of joy and love in your body.

So Smile!

Smile when you are waking up in the morning, and Smile when you are in bed at night drifting into sleep. And Smile every chance you get during your day.

**Extra Credit:** Smile when you are unhappy, in pain, worried, angry or sad.

What if by sending yourself a smile, you will activate a power that will soften your unhappiness, your pain, your worry, your anger and your sadness?

A smile seems to have the magical power to brighten one's day – so brighten someone else's day by smiling at everyone you encounter – and watch your own day brighten up!

## Intention – Choosing What You Want In Life

What are your intentions for your life? Spend a few minutes every day in quiet reflection asking: "What do I want in my life, and what do I want to experience this day?"

You might answer: "I want to experience Love, Joy, Abundance, Gratitude, Grace and Adventure."

Every morning set your intentions (write your intentions for the day in your journal), and let go of *how* they might show up in your life.

Set your intentions for the week, month and year by thoughtfully composing your goals in your journal.

## Attention – Keep Your Eye On The Prize

**Whatever you focus on, Grows:** This is an Eternal Law of Nature, just like gravity.

- ❖ When you keep your attention on Love – Love grows.
- ❖ When you keep your attention on Joy – Joy grows.
- ❖ When you keep your attention on Abundance – Abundance grows.
- ❖ When you keep your attention on Adventure – watch out!
- ❖ When you keep your attention on pain, lack, loneliness and sadness – well, you can guess what grows.

Your attention is very powerful, so tap into this power and use it for your highest good and for the highest good of those in your life.

You will blossom in this direction by getting rid of your TV and also by letting go of any friends who are keeping you down.

**Being in the question, ask yourself:**

 ❖ What does it feel like when I put my attention on Love?
 ❖ What does it feel like when I put my attention on Joy?
 ❖ What does it feel like when I put my attention on Abundance?
 ❖ What does it feel like when I put my attention on Adventure?
 ❖ What does it feel like when I put my attention on Gratitude?
 ❖ What does it feel like when I put my attention on Beauty?

## Walking The Gentle Path

What if your Life can become more enjoyable by simply walking a Gentle Path? What if the gifts of Life are easier to receive when you walk through life with Joy in your heart, sweetness on your lips, gentleness in your steps, thankfulness in your eyes, graciousness in your Soul and Love in your Being? What if Love will come to you with more grace and ease by moving through Life – Being Joy, Being Sweetness, Being Gentle, Being Thankful, Being Gracious and Being Love?

## Make It Fun – Make It Social

**Start a *For The Love Of Joy Club*:** Create a *For The Love Of Joy Club* by finding 4 to 10 people who are interested in bringing more Joy into their lives through this program. Come together each day, at a prearranged time, to review each person's progress from the day before and set goals for the day ahead. Have all the members of the club pair up with another member to act as a *For The Love Of Joy Club* Buddy. *For The Love Of Joy Club* Buddies can offer additional one-on-one support to each other. Enjoy the friendship and support that naturally comes from working together.

**Online *For The Love Of Joy Club*:** Create an online *For The Love Of Joy Club* by bringing together a group of your friends on Facebook, or you can start a *For the Love Of Joy Club* by developing a Meetup. Have your group meet online every day, at a prescheduled time, with the agenda of supporting each member in the group by reviewing their prior day's progress and setting goals for the day ahead. This group may also offer a one-on-one buddy for more personal support. At the completion of the 30 days, you may want to celebrate together in Hawaii or Italy!

The only requirements for membership into the *For The Love Of Joy Club* are for each person to have a copy of this book, *For The Love Of Joy!*, and to commit to fully participating in the 30-day program.

# A Global Moment Of Joy

*One Billion People Coming Together Daily*
*Helping To Create A More Joyful And Peaceful World*

## www. GlobalMomentOfJoy.com

At 12 noon each day, spend a few minutes in Joy, Love and Gratitude. This is a fun way to raise feelings of Joy in yourself, while simultaneously raising the level of Joy in the world. So spend a few minutes in silent Joy at noon everyday, feeling into all that you are grateful for and all that you Love. Send *Love* and *Healing* to a friend who is in pain or to a nation whose citizens are hurting – such as the people living in the Middle East – to help create a more peaceful world.

**Joy in Motion – Taking Action:** Think of ways to bring more Joy into your life and into the life of someone else such as a member of your family, a friend or someone who could use a little more Joy in his/her life, then go and make it happen. Each day, search for ways that you can bring one new Joy into your life and into the life of another. If you are out to lunch with friends ask them to talk about the Joys in their lives, how they can bring more Joy into their lives and into the lives of others. Spread the Joy!

**Be a Joy Ambassador:** Share *A Global Moment of Joy* with your friends and family and with everyone in your social media circle, and encourage them to join in on the fun.

The goal of a Joy Ambassador is to help raise the level of Joy in all life on earth, by having millions of people in each time zone around the world, engaging in *A Global Moment of Joy*. Think of the power of One Billion people coming together every day in Joy, Love and Gratitude.

## The Power of Social Media – Spreading the Joy to One Billion People Around the World

Let's say you invite 100 of your friends to be Joy Ambassadors = 100.

...They invite 100 of their friends = 10,000

...Then the 10,000 invite 100 of their friends = 1,000,000

...Then the 1,000,000 invite 100 of their friends = 100,000,000

...And then the 100,000,000 invite 10 of their friends = **One Billion People bringing Joy, Love and Gratitude into the World!!!**

So help spread the word and be part of creating a more Peaceful and Joyful world.

Learn more at: **www.GlobalMomentOfJoy.com**

## Gaining Wisdom And Clear Intuition

What if Wisdom combined with clear Intuition will bring you inner knowledge that will lead to more happiness and success in life? Wisdom and Intuition come from meditation, quiet reflection, being in the company of someone who is intuitive and wise, reading inspiring books, and by learning from, reflecting on and being with life's experiences.

**Action combined with Wisdom and a Clear Intuition gives you Power! Power to create a more Joyous, Loving and Successful Life!**

# Truth

What if Truth makes you feel lighter, whereas lies make you feel heavier?

What if by living your Truth (that which makes you feel lighter), you begin to see more Joy, Love and Magnificence flow into your life?

This tool may be helpful when making life-decisions: When a choice feels light, you may want to move forward with confidence, and when a choice feels heavy, you may want to pause and reassess.

# Stepping Out Of Your Smallness

Step out of self-pity, blame, entitlement, self-absorption, weakness and smallness.

# Stepping Into Your Power

Step into Taking Responsibility, Respect for oneself and Respect for others, Clarity, Appreciation, Freedom, Wisdom, Courage, Confidence, Expansion, Brilliance and Power!

# The Goal

The Goal of this book is to guide and inspire you to take action that will bring more Joy and Love into your Life. By following the protocol, you may see improvements in all areas of your life including relationships, finance, health and an overall sense of personal well-being.

As stated before, there are no guarantees in life, and there is no guarantee that at the conclusion of this book your life will be bliss and blossoms.

The first three days alone, however, will noticeably help you move your life in a positive direction:

Day 1, **Self-Love**: Every drop of Self-Love you bring into your Being will give you a greater sense of well-being, will put a smile on your face and joy in your heart.

Day 2, **Shake Your Body**: This section is designed to get your heart beating, your lungs and cells oxygenated and your body moving – to enhance your feelings of well-being and improved health.

Day 3, **Good Vibrations**: Today you will be dancing in the morning and singing in the shower, for where there are good vibrations, there is Joy.

## Quantifying Your Progress

It is helpful for you to see your progress as you move through this program. At the beginning and end of each day, reflect in your journal upon how you are feeling, and give yourself a number from 1 to 10: 1 being Deep in the Mud to 10 Feeling the Joy.

## Celebration

It is very important to celebrate every new Joy in your life, both small and big. Celebrate a bonus at work, a great meal – every meal! …a beautiful sunset, a smiling baby, a new blossom in your garden, a new friend or a new love.

Get up and celebrate your Joys by dancing and singing. Create your own special Celebration Dance and Song. Sing along with "Happy" or "Celebrate" or the 1980s tune, "Dance to the Music," or create your own version of musical happiness.

When you celebrate your Joys with Joy, this tells your body, your brain, your subconscious and the Universe, "I want more of this!"

Create or choose two types of Celebration Dance Songs: a quiet one for when you are in public, and a loud one for when you are alone.

**Loud Celebration:** When you are alone – let it rip! Grab a drum, a bell, or a horn, and dance around the room singing "I'm So Happy, I'm So Happy," or any song of your creation or choosing.

**Quiet Celebration:** For celebrating when you are in public, picture a party going on, do a thumb or toe dance or send big smiles to others.

**Being in the question, ask yourself:** "What Joy can I celebrate today?"

# Challenges

We all have challenges, whether they involve family, finances, health or slow traffic. What if every time a challenge comes your way, you embrace it and even approach it with a smile? What if you sent love to every challenge and to the one who is having the challenge (including yourself) no matter how big or small? What if by sending love to the challenge, it gets smaller? I am not suggesting that you love the challenge, but rather that you *send* love *to* the challenge. This is like shining light in the darkness and seeing the darkness turn to light. What if the more love you send, the fewer challenges arise?

What if, as you venture through this book, you gain skills and insights that give you the power and vision to move through your challenges with more Grace and Ease, and what if life brings you fewer and lighter challenges? These are the goals of this 30-day adventure program.

# Enliven

Love Enlivens Love, Joy Enlivens Joy, Trust Enlivens Trust and Beauty Enlivens Beauty . . .

Stress Enlivens stress, pain Enlivens pain, sadness Enlivens sadness and shame Enlivens shame . . .

*What do you choose to Enliven?*

# Put Yourself First

**Yes, Put Yourself First:** Feel into how it feels to Put Yourself First. How does it feel to take a full day to pamper YOU – taking a long, warm, scented bath, taking a nap in the middle of the day, saying *no* to do something you don't really want to do?

Every building needs a strong foundation to function at its highest capacity. By Putting Yourself First, you are nourishing your body, emotions, mind and soul, which allows you to function at the top of your game with joy, love and power.

What if you could Put Yourself First as you gracefully take care of life's responsibilities: Much like putting on your own oxygen mask first and then helping others?!

# Being Joy!

*Pause for a moment. Take some slow relaxing breaths, relax into what it would feel like to:*

*Stop seeking Joy – Be Joy*
*Stop seeking Love – Be Love*
*Stop seeking Abundance – Be Abundance*
*Stop seeking Vitality – Be Vitality*
*Stop seeking Understanding – Be Understanding*
*Stop seeking Peace – Be Peace…*
*Stop seeking Forgiveness – Be Forgiveness*
*Stop seeking Grace – Be Grace*
*Stop seeking God's Love – Be God's Love*

*So Be Joy!*
*Be Love!*
*Be Abundance!*
*Be Vitality!*
*Be Understanding!*
*Be Peace!*
*Be Forgiveness!*

*Be Grace!*
*Be Gods' Love!!!*

# Lighten Up – Have Fun!

What if life could be fun? What if every day brought with it laughter–worthy situations, along with friends to share the laughter? What if you could fly through life with a lighter step, a lighter heart and a lighter mind?

What if you could lighten up by 10 percent, 20 percent, 40 percent or even 80 percent? What if you could bring more light into yourself and into everyone and every situation you encounter?

Feel the pure Joy of having your body, mind, emotions, thoughts, deeds and heart overflowing with Light!

As you move through the next 30 days, choose to experience life in a more fun-loving way. By practicing the 30 programs in this book, you will naturally begin to glow as you move through life.

# Patience

Wouldn't it be wonderful if this book came with a magic wand for you to use to instantly fill your life with Love, Joy, Health and Abundance? In a sense, each of the daily programs and exercises found in this book *do* possess magic that will empower you to let go of anger and fear and move into Love and Joy. If you can be patient with yourself, have faith in the process, and keep your eye on the goal, the magic will unfold day by day. A bit of patience is required.

**Being in the question - Take a moment to feel into:**

❖ What would it feel like to have Patience and to fully Trust?

❖ What would it feel like to hold the goals of Love, Joy, Health and Abundance and to patiently watch as they gracefully unfold into your life?

# Keep It Simple

What if one of the fastest ways to bring more Joy into your life is to simplify?

**Simplify Your Home** – Organize your home to both look beautiful and to help you to be efficient. You may want to research Feng Shui – Feng Shui is a Chinese philosophical system for harmonizing your home's environment – to enliven peace, health and prosperity. Get rid of any clutter by using the *Six Month Rule*, if you have not used an item in the last six months you might think about donating it.

**Simplify Your Relationships** – Life is much more fun when your relationships are light and rich.

**Simplify Your Finances** – The best ways to simplify your finances are:

1. Spend less than your income
2. Save
3. Be Grateful
4. Be Generous
5. As you go through your day look for ways to lessen your outflow of money and to increase your inflow
6. Look for ways to simplify your life by down-sizing

In Day-17, *Abundance*, you will delve deeper into the subject of money and wealth.

**Simplify Yourself** – Move forward with everything that makes you feel expansive and let go of, or get out of the way of, everything that makes you feel contracted. Keep It Simple.

# Life Is A Process

There is no finish line here that reads: "Joy, Love and Beauty." It is not likely that you will be flowing in the bliss of Joy, Love and Beauty 24/7. (If you are, please give me a call).

> As long as you are moving *closer* to Joy
> and bringing *more* Love and Beauty
> into your Life, you are as good as Gold!

## Love

What would it feel like to truly Love Yourself, to truly Love Your Life and to truly Love Others? What if, over time, by sending Love to your Heart and really feeling into that Love, much healing can occur, and Love and Abundance can naturally flow into your Life with Grace and Ease? What if *I Love You*, spoken out loud or softly to yourself will call forth a Universal Power? What if by invoking this Universal Power, you will awaken within yourself Joy and Love on the physical, emotional and spiritual levels? What if *I Love You* could be your magic wand in Life? What if you could bring more Light, Love and Joy into your Life, one *I Love You* at a time?

## Warning

This book contains exercises that may bring a smile to your face, more joy to your heart and increased peace of mind. You may find yourself liking yourself more and LOVING LIFE.

As with any new physical activity or diet, it is best to talk with your doctors. I recommend that you show your doctors this book (or gift them a copy), and have them be an active part of your support team.

As you proceed, move into each day's program with Ease and Joy; straining on any level is not constructive to your progress.

# How To Use This Book

By including the following programs into your daily living, you will feel more Joy and Love in your Life at the conclusion of this book.

Each day's program is very powerful and, if sincerely applied, will help to move your life forward. From Day 1 – Self-Love – you will be immersed in the warm ocean of Loving Yourself completely.

Move through this day, and the following days, in a gentle way, being mindful that you are on an adventure: Make it fun and enjoyable, while keeping an affectionate eye on your goal of increasing Love and Joy in your Life.

These programs are designed to support you. It is best to take each day in order (no jumping ahead to Day 19 – Romance). Each day's program is specially designed to give support to the following day. So get into the flow, have fun and proceed with Ease and Grace.

Selfie: Take a photo of yourself and adhere it to page viii. At the conclusion, on day 30, take another photo of yourself and adhere it below your starting photo. Do you see a bigger smile in the new photo?

Each day you will be given **Living Words** such as Courage, Certainty, Power, Love and Gratitude. Feel into the essence of these words, and infuse them into your entire Being as you go through your day. Feel free to choose additional words that bring Power, Joy and Love into your Life.

Bring out your playful nature as you venture through the next 30 days. Put your serious side in your back pocket, and jump into the excitement of this new adventure.

You are now ready to save your Life: Sign and date the commitment pledge on the next page, put a smile on your face and get ready for a hearty dose of Self-Love!

# Getting Started

It is strongly recommended that you include the following measures as you start this 30-day adventure:

**Keep a Daily Journal** – Each morning write your intentions for the day in your journal; and each evening add your accomplishments and what you are grateful for.

**Eat Healthy** – Increase your intake of greens and water (filtered or bottled – with no chlorine or fluoride).

**Qigong/Yoga** – Take a Qigong or Yoga class from a certified instructor. Qigong (pronounced Chi Gong) and Yoga are gentle forms of exercise that greatly improve your health on all levels: Emotional, physical and mental.

**Healthy Sleep** – Each night it is best to have all electronics – (TV, computer, telephone) – turned off by 8:00 p.m., and be in bed before 10:00 p.m. (This is a suggestion for optimum results, and not a strict rule).

**Smile** – Smiling raises your body's endorphins, so Smile – especially when you do not feel like smiling.

**Your Best Self** – Bring your best self to this 30-day journey!

# Making The Commitment

Here is the moment of Truth.

Are you ready to do all that is necessary to move your Life into more Love and Joy?

If you are, please sign your name **(Boldly)** and date this pledge of personal commitment:

**I** _____

**hereby Commit to My Joy, Love, Health, Life and to fully accomplishing each day's program to the best of my ability. I further commit to being kind to myself throughout this program.**

---

### Signed and Dated

*Please note: If at any time you feel that a daily program is not in line with your moral principles, you may skip that program.*

**Are you ready to get started?**

If so, put a smile on your face and let's dive into Day 1: Self-Love!

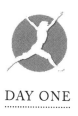

# Self-Love

Wʰᵃᵗ if there is a Universal Power that you can tap into, which will bring more harmony into your life? What if Love combined with this Universal Power will naturally fill your life with more Joy, Health, Abundance and Self-Love?

The goal of Day 1 is to shine Self-Love into every cell of your body, into every emotion, into every thought, into every action. For where there is authentic Self-Love – Love without reservation – your true self unfolds, your trivial woes lose their potency and Joy and Confidence naturally develop.

## The Highest Form of Self-Love

This is not a self centered, Ego-driven love. **This is Love's highest and fullest expression of knowing who you are, celebrating your Magnificence, being thankful, and living in your full Glory. A Love where you are in the highest service to your Self, service to God, and service to God's creation.**

Today you will start by sending *I Love Yous* to every experience, every thought, every feeling… everything you see – especially to any pains in your body.

It is best to say "I Love You" out loud (if you are in public, say it to yourself) with your right hand on your chest to feel the vibrations of the words. Sing "I Love You" as you would to a two-year-old baby.

Every *I Love You* that you send into yourself, or out to others, will help to change the chemistry of your body from pain to Joy, from dis-ease to Health, from bondage to Flow. Visualize every *I Love You* entering and lighting up your 64 trillion cells and cleaning house.

At first you may think: "This is silly" or "I am in such pain and anger, how can I send *I Love Yous*?" This is the time when you must recommit to the 30-day program and JUST DO IT! You get extra credit for saying "I Love You" with a big smile.

This is a very powerful process. Every time you say "I Love You," it acts like a reboot. When a negative thought arises, send it an *I Love You*. The goal here is to clear out old thought patterns and replace them with Love.

With every *I Love You*, you are invoking the most powerful force in the Universe. This is the Love that created you, that created all life on earth – the sun, our solar system, our galaxy and the entire Universe. This is more than just a soft and warm feeling; it is the power of the Creator of the Universe, moving through you. Grab it, Enjoy it, Feel it – Live It!

As with any new habit, your *I Love You* mantras will get easier and become more effective over time.

## Loving Your Body –
## Tender Loving Care for Your Body

You are a walking, talking, eating and digesting miracle. Every minute – 24/7 – your body is conducting millions of intricate and precise actions that keep you alive. You have around 64 trillion cells, and each of these cells functions in perfect harmony to keep you alive. What would your life be like if your stomach stopped working, or your kidneys, liver, heart, eyes, brain, feet or lungs no longer functioned? As you go through your day, send *I Loves Yous* to your body in appreciation for the miracle that it is.

## I LOVE YOU

The following activities are simple, yet very powerful.

Sing "I Love You" to your Heart for three minutes when you wake up, while lying in bed, and for three minutes before you go to sleep. Hold your hand over your heart and feel your chest vibrate as you sing "I Love You" to yourself. Feel the Love and smile.

As you go through your day send *I Love Yous* to every experience, every thought, every feeling and everything you see.

Send *I Love Yous* to any part of the body that is in pain and to any fear, anger, rage, guilt or shame.

To my pain – *I Love You*
To my sadness  – *I Love You*
To my rage – *I Love You*
To my guilt – *I Love You*
To my shame – *I Love You*
To my body – *I Love You*
To my heart – *I Love You*
To my mind – *I Love You*
To my beauty – *I Love You*
To my Self – *I Love You*


## Journal Your Intentions for the Day

My intention for today: I intend to feel and be Powerful, Joyful, Courageous and Loving towards myself and to act in a Loving way towards all that I experience today.


## Learn to Let Go of Anger

Become a Master of Self-Love, and watch your life shine in miraculous ways. This is a lifelong process. Be easy on yourself as you explore bringing more love and joy into your life.

There is a story about a tribe in Africa that has mastered the art of capturing monkeys. First, a hunter would attach a basket to a tree. Next, he would put the monkey's favorite food in the basket. The basket has a hole in the top just big enough for the monkey to put its hand in to grab the food. The hole is too small for the monkey to get his hand out of the basket with the food. As hard as the monkey tries, it cannot get its hand out of the basket. The harder the monkey tries to free its hand with the food, the more exhausted it becomes. When the hunter returns, the monkey will not release its hand from the food to free itself and the monkey is easily captured.

Are you holding on to something that is keeping you stuck in the basket... or in the mud?

Are you holding on to anger, stress, fear, resentment, jealousy, sadness and darkness?

What would happen if you just opened your hand and released it all – all the anger, all the stress, all the fear, all the resentment...the jealousy, the sadness, the darkness?

Just let go! It is impossible to be Love when you are holding on to anger and fear, sadness and darkness.

## Love – Love – Love
### *Swimming in the Sea of Love*

What if Love is like an unbounded Ocean full of expansion, power, serenity and beauty?

The ocean is perfectly calm in its natural state – it is an unbounded field of silence and emptiness, a Field of All Possibilities. Like the ocean, when you are in this state of perfect calm, the true power of Love is at your command.

It is when the winds of life blow that waves appear on the surface of the ocean. These waves carry the feelings of Love's arousal, joy, bliss, unity and sensuality; in addition to sadness, separation, jealousy and fear.

So Be In Love. Spend a few minutes every morning when you first wake up and again at night just before you fall asleep, floating in this Unbounded Sea of Love. Close your eyes, take four slow, deep breaths, and lovingly fall into the warm and soft feelings of Love. Feel the Warmth, the Serenity, the Power and the Joy of Pure Love!

**The following are very effective exercises for increasing feelings of Joy and for freeing unwanted emotions.**

**Releasing Anger** – Clench your hands into fists as tightly as you can. Hold this position for 30 seconds while thinking of your anger and fear. After 30 seconds, thrust open your hands and release your anger and fear. Doing this exercise a few times each day will help release the cellular memory of your anger.

**I Love You Hula** – Start your morning with the *I Love You Hula*. Stand with your feet two feet apart, and your hands on your hips. Now slowly rotate your hips around like you are whirling a hula-hoop. Rotate nine times to the right and nine times to the left while you are singing *I Love Yous* to yourself. This will stimulate your first chakra (Personal Survival), second chakra (Sensuality), and third chakra (Personal Power). Check out Google and YouTube to learn more about chakras.

It is best to perform the *I Love You Hula* outside, facing the morning sun.

**Love Hug** – Anytime you need a little more happiness, give yourself a Love Hug. Lovingly wrap your arms around yourself while sweetly sending your entire being *I Love Yous*.

**A Sweetheart Engenders a Sweet-Heart** – A warm embrace with your Sweetheart in the morning, at night and throughout the day is a wonderful way to enliven the joy of Self-Love in your heart and body.

**Be Love** – Today, and for the rest of your life, Go for the Love! Fill yourself with Love, ignite your heart with Love, encase every thought and word with Love, immerse your entire Being in Love, and then Go and Shine Your Love into the World.

If you need a little extra help, spend time with babies and puppies; they are pure Love and Joy.

**Being in the question – Take a moment to feel into:**

- ❖ What would it feel like to Love Myself deeper than anyone ever has before?
- ❖ What would it feel like to swim in the unbounded Ocean of Love?
- ❖ What would it feel like to live in the calmness of the unbounded Ocean of Love?
- ❖ What would it feel like to master the power of True Love?
- ❖ What would it feel like to fully trust the Universe to Lovingly Support Me?
- ❖ What would it feel like to fully Love My Life?
- ❖ What would it feel like to fully Enjoy My Uniqueness?
- ❖ What would it feel like to fully to expand My Beauty, My Creativity and My God Given Talents?
- ❖ What would it feel like to walk through life with a Happy Heart?
- ❖ What would it feel like to fully Shine?
- ❖ What would it feel like to Be Love?

**Living Words:** Love, Power, Grace, Trust, Self-Love, Unbounded, Sweetness and Hugs.

*This is a subtle truth:*
*whatever you love, you are.*

—Rumi

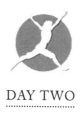

# Shake Your Body

Today you will enliven your being on all levels – physical, mental, emotional and spiritual. You are a physical being – and when your heart is beating fast with life-giving blood, your lungs are inspired with life-giving oxygen, your brain is nourished, and your limbs are moving – you will feel happier, healthier and stronger, think more clearly, and have a greater sense of personal well-being.

**Be sure to talk with your doctor about adding new physical activities to your daily routine.**

The goal here is to have fun and be energized at the same time. Identify an aerobic activity that you want to add to your life. There is a full list below. Choose one or two activities and sign up for a class. Whether you choose dance, yoga, tennis, or Tai Chi, activities are much more fun when done with friends, and when you are at a level of proficiency. So grab some friends and sign up for a class.

It is important that you schedule the activity into your life at least two times per week, preferably more. Have fun while you are dancing, running or doing yoga. Never strain your body or over-commit. If you are smiling while you are doing the activity, you are doing it right.

**Dance:** Dancing will keep you young! Take a dance class such as swing, tango or waltz, and go out dancing at least once every week. (If you are in a relationship, encourage your mate to join you).

**Yoga and Qigong:** Take a Yoga or Qigong class. Yoga and Qigong are exceptionally good for your heart, body and soul. Both activities have been proven to help reduce stress, strengthen your body and improve your health.

**Swim:** Swimming works the entire body and helps to get more oxygen into your cells. Just being in the water makes you feel fresh, happy and clean.

**Tennis:** Tennis has it all: It is social, it is fun, it is aerobic and hitting the ball is a great way to release anger and frustration.

**Walk:** Take a walk in nature, in the woods, along a lake or on an ocean beach. Enjoy nature's beauty as you breathe in the fresh, life-giving air that will enliven your body and soul.

**Create a Vegetable Garden:** Be in the joy of growing your own food, getting your hands in the dirt and watching your garden grow.

**Shake Your Body:** Run, ski, bike skate, kick-box, belly dance, row, play volleyball or basketball, skip and do Zumba.

**Being in the question – Take a moment to feel into:**

❖ What would it feel like to fully Love My Body?
❖ What would it feel like to Sparkle?
❖ What would it feel like to be Vibrant?
❖ What would it feel like to feel Exhilarated?
❖ What would it feel like to be in Perfect Health?
❖ What would it feel like to be Physically and Mentally Strong?

**Living Words:** Love, Strength, Health, Vibrant, Wellbeing, Action, Exhilarated, Sparkle, Flow and Alive.

*Whenever we manage to love without expectations, calculations, negotiations, we are indeed in heaven.*

# —Rumi

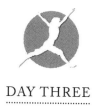

# Good Vibrations

Quantum science shows that everything is vibration: from the food you eat to the clothes you wear, from the color of your fingernail polish to your thoughts and emotions.

## Vibration of Love Chart

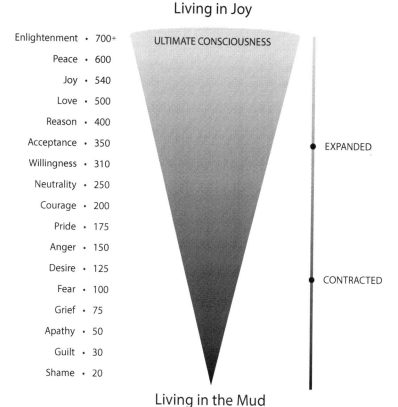

Living in Joy

| | | |
|---|---|---|
| Enlightenment · 700+ | ULTIMATE CONSCIOUSNESS | |
| Peace · 600 | | |
| Joy · 540 | | |
| Love · 500 | | |
| Reason · 400 | | |
| Acceptance · 350 | | EXPANDED |
| Willingness · 310 | | |
| Neutrality · 250 | | |
| Courage · 200 | | |
| Pride · 175 | | |
| Anger · 150 | | |
| Desire · 125 | | |
| Fear · 100 | | CONTRACTED |
| Grief · 75 | | |
| Apathy · 50 | | |
| Guilt · 30 | | |
| Shame · 20 | | |

Living in the Mud

What if feeling sad, lonely, fearful and depressed is a result of choosing certain foods, clothes, colors, thoughts and emotions that vibrate at a lower level?

What if you can feel more joy by choosing to feel abundant, safe, expansive, confident; and also by choosing foods, clothes, thoughts and emotions that vibrate at higher levels?

Take a look at the Vibration of Love Chart. Where are you currently holding? (Vibrating between 20-150: anger, fear, shame)? Where would you like to be holding? (Vibrating above 500: love, peace, joy)? What if the choice is yours?

Today, and for the rest of your life, choose higher-vibrating thoughts, emotions, food, clothes and friends. The goal here is to vibrate at 500 or above.

## Techniques for Raising Your Vibration

**Essential Oils:** One of the fastest ways to raise your vibration is to wear essential oils. Essential oils are gifts from nature that have amazing healing, rejuvenating, and uplifting abilities.

You will receive feelings of Euphoria and Joy from wearing sweet orange or rose essential oils. (Rose has the highest vibration of all the essential oils). Always use high-quality organic oils.

Apply sweet orange or rose first thing in the morning and reapply it throughout your day and evening, as you would a perfume or cologne. Place some oil under your nose and on your temples. It is best to dilute your essential oils in a base oil such as grape-seed oil or extra-virgin olive oil. Learn more by Googling: Essential Oils and Aromatherapy.

**Singing in the Shower, in the Car, at Work, with Your Family:**
Sing your favorite songs like you are a Rock Star! And hum vowel sounds while you are taking your morning shower. Humming the vowel sounds will raise your emotional vibration and will physically enliven you by pulsating the vibrations in your chest. With a smile on your face, put your hands on your chest while you hum—HA, HAE, HE, HO, HU. Humming also helps your body to loosen and release stress and other negative, trapped emotions.

**Emotional Freedom Technique (EFT):** Emotional Freedom Technique is a very powerful tool for letting go of lower emotions such as shame, guilt, grief, fear and anger, while bringing more expansive emotions such as Love, Joy and Peace into your life. EFT is a process of using your fingers to tap on specific acupressure points on your body. This tapping helps to open up trapped emotions in your body, allowing healing to begin. Emotional Freedom Technique is easy to learn and can be done anywhere and at any time. To learn more about EFT, check out the excellent videos on YouTube or you may seek out a certified EFT practitioner in your area.

**Beauty:** Beauty is all around you. It is waiting for you to take notice of it, to relax into its Joy and to be truly thankful for it. Seek to find and appreciate Beauty as you walk through your day. Start with the beautiful *you*! When you arise each morning, lovingly gaze at yourself in the mirror and say, "Hello, Beautiful!" For an extra-high vibe-ing experience, playfully give yourself some *I Love Yous* for a full minute, as you appreciate the miracle in the mirror… and just watch your life change!

**Wear Bright Colors:** Wear colors that uplift your spirit.

**Eat Healthy Food:** Eat foods that are healthful and alive. Be mindful when you are eating by thoroughly tasting, enjoying and feeling gratitude with every bite.

**Be with Happy Friends:** Choose friends who are living happy and fulfilling lives. Say good-bye to friends who bring you down.

**Smile:** A heartfelt smile will always bring a little joy to your heart, so smile often.

## Daily Routine

The following Daily Routine is designed to bring more happiness, health and well-being into your life. Embrace this Daily Routine with Grace. Ease into it. As you walk through your day, add your own ideas for enriching your life, health and happiness.

# Morning

When you first wake up, while in bed:

**1. Start Your Day With Joy, Gratitude and Love!** When you first wake up, with your eyes closed, feel into a few moments of pure Gratitude, as you count your many blessings. Then, feel into all of the Joys that you would like to experience in the next 24 hours. Smile as you feel the joyfulness in your heart and your body the joyfulness of all the Yums and Wows that you desire to have today.

**Three minutes of "I Love Yous."** Put your right hand over your heart, close your eyes and take slow, deep breaths in and out while singing "I Love You" to your heart or to any part of your body that needs attention. Relax and let yourself feel into the euphoric warmth of Love.

**Prayer before rising:** You may offer your own prayer, or you may say: "This is the day that the Lord has made, I will rejoice and be happy therein. Dear God, what Love, Joy, Beauty and Peace can I bring into the world today?"

**2. Journal your intentions for the day.** Write in your journal and say out loud or to yourself: "Today I intend to Love Myself. Today I intend to bring Beauty into my Life. Today I intend to bring Joy into my Life."

**3. Happy Dance!** Pop out of bed dancing a Happy Dance, as if you just scored a winning touchdown. Feel into something you deeply desire in your life (deeper love, perfect health, great wealth, a romantic trip to Italy!). Feel as if you are experiencing this deeper love, this perfect health, this great wealth and this romance in Italy right now, and smile as you start your day with a fun, Happy Dance.

**4. Stretch.** Get out of bed like a lion and greet the day with 5-10 minutes of exercise (Qigong and yoga are perfect for starting your day). Qigong is a very gentle and easy form of exercise that can bring healing to your body, joy to your heart, balance to your emotions and power to your soul. Learn more about Qigong via Google and YouTube.

**5. Singing in the rain.** Sing and hum in the shower with a smile.

**6. Add a little rose or sweet orange essential oil** to your body playfully and sensually! If you like, add your essential oil to a base oil such as grape-seed or sesame-seed, and give yourself a loving full-body massage!

**7. Morning Meditation.**

**8. Eat a healthy breakfast.** Eat slowly and mindfully, enjoying each bite while feeling thankful for the food.

**9. Leave for work 10 minutes early.** This way you will not be stressed if you find yourself in slow traffic.

**As You Move Through Your Day:**

- ❖ Send *I Love Yous* to your beautiful self, knowing that every "I Love You" is like a drop of sparkling water washing the mud from your heart and the stress from every cell.
- ❖ Look for the Beauty, Love and Joy.
- ❖ Hum and Sing – Humming and Singing bring Joy to the Heart and helps to release pain and sorrow on an emotional and physical level.


# Afternoon

**1. A Global Moment of Joy:** Join with potentially One Billion People from around the world at 12-noon everyday to spend a few minutes in Joy, Love and Gratitude. This is a fun way to raise feelings of Joy in you, while simultaneously raising the level of Joy in the world. So spend a few minutes in Joy at noon everyday in silent Joy, feeling into all that you are grateful for and all that you Love, and send *Love* and *Healing* to a friend who is hurting or to a nation whose citizens are hurting–such as the people of the Middle East–to help create a more peaceful world.

**Joy in Action:** Think of ways to bring more Joy into your life and into the life of someone else and then go and make it happen. Everyday, look for ways to bring a new joy into your life and into the life of another. If you are out to lunch with friends, ask them to talk about their Joys and Loves, and how they can bring more Joy into their lives and into the lives of others. Spread the Joy!

**Be a Joy Ambassador:** Share *A Global Moment of Joy* with everyone in your social media circles and encourage them to join with potentially millions of people in each time zone to bring an infusion of Joy, Love and Gratitude to the world everyday at noon. Help spread the word and be part of creating a more Peaceful and Joyful world. Check out A Global Moment of Joy at: www.GlobalMomentOfJoy.com

**2. Healthy lunch with friends**

**3. Enjoy Essential Oils**

**4. Shake your body – Swim, Dance and Yoga . . .**

**5. Afternoon Meditation**

## Night

**1. Healthy dinner—Being mindful and thankful for the food.**

**2. Sensuously apply some Rose or Sweet Orange oil.**

**3. By 8:00 p.m. all electrics are off** (TV, computer, telephone).

**4. By 10:00 p.m. in bed.**

**5. Journal about your joys and successes of the day, and compose your desired joys and successes for tomorrow.**

**6. Set your intention for your sleep and dreams:** I intend to have a restful and restorative night of sleep with dreams that are Adventurous, Loving, Joyful and Healing.

**Being in the question – Take a moment to feel into:**

- ❖ What would it feel like to fully be Happy?
- ❖ What would it feel like to Live in the Vibration of Love?
- ❖ What would it feel like to Live in the Vibration of Abundance?
- ❖ What would it feel like to bring more Joy, Love and Peace to the world?

**Living Words:** Love, Joy, Peace, Trust, Energy, Action, Power and Good Vibrations.

## Healing Music

The following musicians have a worldwide reputation for composing and playing inspirational music that elevates your physiological vibrations, enabling you to feel happier, healthier and more peaceful.

**Barry Goldstein: www.BarryGoldsteinMusic.com.** Barry has a very special talent of infusing the Universal Power of Love into his music.

**Jim Oliver: www.JimOliverMusic.com.** Jim fuses healing sound with color to uplift one's body and soul.

**Jonathan Goldman: www.HealingSounds.com.** Jonathan has a large selection of courses and music downloads that will open you to higher levels of Joy and Healing.

**Steve Halpern: www.SteveHalpern.com.** Steve's special music will offer you vibrations that are relaxing, healing, meditative, and will help to bring on restful sleep.

## Vibration Of Love Chart

Dr. David Hawkins MD, PhD ingeniously created the Vibration Of Love Chart that is pictured on page 31. This chart measures the vibrational frequencies of human emotions from 20 megahertz (shame) to 700 megahertz (Enlightenment). The goal is to be at 500 megahertz (Love or above).

*Keep on knocking 'til the joy*
*inside opens a window—look*
*to see who's there.*

## —Rumi

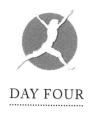

DAY FOUR

# Composing Your Life Story – Taking Charge of Your Life!

## *Write It Down – Make It Happen!*

Today you will become a Romance author – and *you* are the main love interest.

This is your moment to shine: Write the story of your life starting from this moment, continue on straight through the rest of your life.

Have fun and fill your story with adventure, excitement, mission, love, family, friends, pets and meaningful work that celebrates your gifts and talents. Fill your story with creativity, Italy – or your favorite place to visit – and other details of your life overflowing with Joy.

Purchase a beautiful journal, and with Joy in your heart and a Smile on your face, start composing your life's story!

**Bringing Your Life Story To Life!** Now that you have composed your Fun, Joyous, Loving, Adventurous and Luscious Life, go and LIVE IT!

**This Is Your Life** – All that is required is for you to put a smile in your heart and focus your full attention on living a rewarding, loving and meaningful life.

**Living Words:** Adventure, Fun, Command, Home, Family, Marriage, Children, Grandchildren, Great-Grandchildren, Romance, Fortune, Service, Healthy, Gratitude, Creation, Creative, Magnificence, Passion, Personal Power, Personal Growth, Spiritual Connection, Fulfillment, Love, Life, Italy and Joy!

**Being in the question – Take a moment to feel into:**

- ❖ What would it feel like to write my Love Story?
- ❖ What would it feel like to Live my Love Story?
- ❖ What would it feel like to fully Let Go?
- ❖ What would it feel like to Create a Magnificent Life?
- ❖ What would it feel like to Live My Magnificent Life?
- ❖ What would it feel like to fully Create Beauty and Joy?
- ❖ What would it feel like to know that all is in perfect right order?

*Everyone has been made for some
particular work and the desire for that
work has been put in every heart.*

## —Rumi

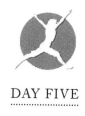

# Passion

What if Passion is the juice that helps to fuel a happy life? What if you can ignite your passions *right now* and by doing so bring more joy into your life?

What if adding the *WOW! Factor* and the *Yum! Factor* into every experience, you will turn on your passions?

## *The WOW! Factor*

The *WOW! Factor* is very simple yet very powerful. The *WOW! Factor* is experiencing life like a three-year-old child, experiencing everything in life with fresh eyes and a sense of wonder and discovery.

What if feeling a WOW! awakens your passions? Go for the WOW! anytime you see a baby, a flower, a mountain, your lover, your hand, your eyes, the eyes of a loved one… and all the magic that life brings your way!

What if by expressing, in a heartfelt way, a *WOW!* either to yourself or out loud, you are not only igniting your passions and expanding your joy, you are telling the Universe: "I want more of this!" And the Universe responds, "Your wish is my command!"?

## *The Yum! Factor*

The *Yum! Factor* is a dynamic and fun way to experience all the sensual joys of life, from eating a delicious meal (any meal) – yum!, to breathing the morning air, to making soft and slow love, to feeling the warm water on your body when showering, to skinny dipping in a warm ocean, to reveling in music that moves you, to enjoying the scent of a red rose, to holding a baby, to receiving or giving a gentle body massage – *Yum!*

When a kitten purrs, that kitten is enjoying the *Yum! Factor*.

Feel into that *yumminess* and express gratitude and a *Yum* every time you are enjoying sensual pleasure. By doing so, the Universe just might shower you with more of the same.

As you move through your day, add the *WOW! Factor* and the *Yum! Factor* as often as you can, and watch your life become more exciting, fun and filled with passion.

Every night before you drift off to sleep, take a few moments to reflect on the *WOWs!* and the *Yums!* you enjoyed earlier that day. Feel into the feeling of each *WOW!* and *Yum!* as you write them down in your journal, with a smile on your face and joy and gratitude in your heart.

In the morning, take a few minutes in silent meditation to set your intentions for the day. Make sure to put in a request for all the *WOWs!* and the *Yums!* you would like to experience in the next 24 hours. Feel your joy as you write your intentions and the *WOWs!* and the *Yums!* for the day in your morning journal.

This may be difficult at first, but in time you may find a new happiness filling your entire Being!

**Being in the question – Take a moment to feel into:**

- ❖ What would it feel like to fully Live My Passion?
- ❖ What would it feel like to be in the *WOW!*?
- ❖ What would it feel like to fully enjoy all the *Yums!* in life?
- ❖ What would it feel like to jump out of bed every morning with Passion and Joy?
- ❖ What would it feel like to jump into bed every night feeling Passion and Joy?
- ❖ What would it feel like to be full of Gratitude?
- ❖ What would it feel like to be fully Trusting?
- ❖ What would it feel like for my entire Being to be immersed in Joy?

**A Good Read:**

*The Passion Test*, created by Chris Attwood and Janet Bray Attwood, **www.ThePassionTest.com**, will provide you with clear, simple and effective techniques to help you recognize your core passions. This will assist you in creating a happy, meaningful and purpose-filled life. Once you identify and live your passions, watch out – life will get very exciting.

**Living Words:** Passion, Joy, Happy, Gratitude, WOW, Yum, Juicy, Alive, Thrilled and Complete.

*Set your life on fire.*
*Seek those who fan your flames.*
—Rumi

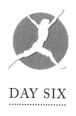

# Living Words

What if all words possess a Life Force? What if your words set the course for your life? What if by choosing words that are uplifting, inspiring, expanding and loving, your life will be more uplifting, inspiring, expanding and loving?

The following is a very powerful technique that will bring the Life Force of words into your emotional, physical and mental Being.

Every morning and as you walk through your day, choose **Living Words** that give you strength and that move you forward in life. Feel into the power of each word as you place them on the triangle or star on your body. (Imagine that the triangle or star is placed on your body as in the images on the next page).

**Bringing Your Words to Life:** Breathe words such as Certain, Capable, Love, Gracious, Power, Generous and Happy into your very essence as you go through your day. With every thought you think, with every word you speak, and with every action you take, be Certain, be Capable, be Love, be Gracious, be Power, be Generous and be Happy. You get extra credit if you can do this with a smile.

Feel free to use **Living Words** of your choosing and to change your **Living Words** at any time to help you glide through life with Power, Joy and Grace.

You may want to start by wearing three **Living Words**, as is seen in the figure on the left. In time you may want to increase your power by wearing six **Living Words** as is shown in the figure on the right.

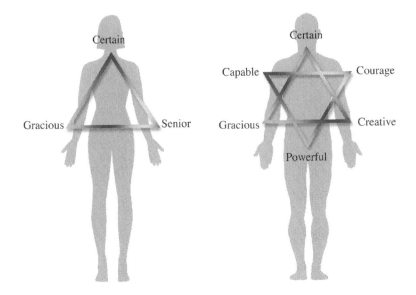

You may choose your own words or use the following:

- ❖ I Am Certain.
- ❖ I Am Capable.
- ❖ I Am Love.
- ❖ I Am Gracious.
- ❖ I Am Powerful.
- ❖ I Am Generous.
- ❖ I Am Happy.
- ❖ I Am Expanding Joy.
- ❖ I Am Radiant Beauty.
- ❖ I Am Brilliant Life.
- ❖ I Am Thankful.

**Being in the question – Take a moment to feel into:**

- ❖ What would it feel like to be Confident, Courageous, Capable, Powerful and Beautiful?
- ❖ What would it feel like to be Loving, Trusting and Fulfilled?
- ❖ What would it feel like to be Gracious, Compassionate and Allowing?

**Living Words:** Capable, Certain, Gracious, Senior, Abundant, Thankful, Alive, Love, Peace, Balance, Harmony, Brilliant, Magnificent, Joy and Fulfilled.

Take a look at **www.MasteringAlchemy.com** to take **Living Words** to a higher level. In addition, this website offers you a full selection of free videos by Jim Self, which will enrich your life.

*Speak a new language so that the world
will be a new world.*

—Rumi

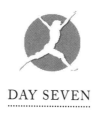

# Friendship
## *Feeling Fully Supported*

The Joys of Life are greatly enhanced when shared with friends and family. This adventure into Joy will be much more fun and successful with good friends, close family members and a support group walking with you.

**FRIENDSHIP:** Find a walking buddy – a two-legged or four-legged kind or both – and go for a walk-and-talk at least once a week.

**Joy Coach:** Invite a close friend or family member to be your Joy Coach. A Joy Coach is a wise, compassionate and trusted person who wants the best for you. Invite your Joy Coach to be there for you however you need her/him to be, as you go through this program and also as you go through life. Meet with your Joy Coach at least once a week. Share with her/him the areas of focus that you are addressing, as well as your goals, and ask for help with anything you need.

**Start a Joy Club:** Create a Joy Club by finding 4 to 10 people who are interested in bringing more Joy into their lives through this program. Every week come together to review each person's progress from the week before and set goals for the week ahead. Have all the members of the club pair up one-on-one with another member to act as a Joy Club Buddy. Joy Club Buddies can offer more personalized support to each other.

**Online Joy Club:** Create an online Joy Club by bringing together a group of your friends on Facebook, or organize a Meetup. Have your group meet online every week at a pre-scheduled time, with the purpose of supporting each member. Review each person's progress from the prior week, and let each share her/his goals for the week ahead. This group may also offer a one-on-one buddy for more personalized support.

The only requirements for membership into the Joy Club are for each person to have a copy of this book, *For The Love Of Joy!*, and to commit to fully participating in the 30-day program.

**Being in the question – Take a moment to feel into:**

- ❖ What would it feel like to be Best Friends with Myself?
- ❖ What would it feel like to have the Support of a Close Friend?
- ❖ What would it feel like to fully Give Friendship?
- ❖ What would it feel like to be fully supported by Life?

**Living Words:** Warmth, Held, Accepting, Support, Feeling Supported, Love, Friendship, Family and Connection.

*Be grateful for whoever comes,*
*because each has been sent as*
*a guide from beyond.*

# —Rumi

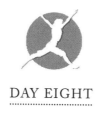

# Putting Yourself First– Time for You to Shine!

### *Being Kind to Yourself: Self-Love, Self-Respect, Self-Acceptance, Self-Esteem, Confidence*

When the sun rises in the morning, all the darkness dissipates and light shines on everyone. So be a Rising Sun and shine your light everywhere you go.

**YES, SHINE!** What if you could help create a better future for yourself, your family and for all life, by putting yourself first, by filling your cup to overflowing, by being kind to yourself and by becoming your own best friend?

What would it feel like to Glow, filled with the light of Love, Joy, Grace, Beauty, Forgiveness, Gratitude, Splendor, Harmony and Generosity? For, it is only when you are full that you can fully give.

From a very early age, many of us are taught that it is best to give to others, which is true. It is wonderful to give to others. The missing piece in that teaching is that we can give more when we have more: We can give more Love when we are Overflowing with Love; we can give more Joy when we are Joyful; we can give better Advice when we have an Abundance of Wisdom; we can give Comfort when we are in Harmony.

As you go through the next 22 days, and for the rest of your life, see yourself gently floating down the river of Self-Love, absorbing Joy, Love, Kindness, Forgiveness, Wisdom and Gratitude along the way.

This is a very special opportunity to fill yourself with light, to the point of overflowing, by pampering yourself while learning how to set boundaries, how to be kind to yourself, and how to enjoy your own company.

1. **Fill your cup** with Sleep, Learning, Growing, Joy, Harmony, Grace and Fulfillment.

2. **Pamper yourself** with Massage, Walks, Nature and Quiet Time.

3. **Set Boundaries** by saying Yes to what feels good and saying No to what does not feel good.

4. **Be Kind to Yourself** by letting go of all negative self-talk. From this point forward, all self-talk will be as if you are talking to your best friend.
   From this point forward, you will take a few moments in your day to compliment yourself.
   As you go through your day, stop and ask Yourself, "What is most Loving to me right now?" Then go and do for Yourself what is Most Loving right now!

5. **Enjoy Your Own Company** by becoming your own best friend. Spend time alone in nature – reading, meditating and in quiet reflection. Relax into feeling happy by being in your own company.

Here are four ways that I am going to bring more Light, Joy and Self-Love into my Life:

1. _____

2. _____

3. _____

4. _____

**Being in the question – Take a moment to feel into:**

- ❖ What is Loving to me right now?
- ❖ What would it feel like to Love Myself?
- ❖ What would it feel like for my cup to be overflowing with Love?
- ❖ What would it feel like to admire Myself?
- ❖ What would it feel like to truly respect Myself?
- ❖ What would it feel like to fully enjoy my own company?
- ❖ What would it feel like to be fully confident?
- ❖ What would it feel like to like Myself?
- ❖ What would it feel like to be happy?

**Living Words:** Kindness, Free, Confident, Liking Myself, Love, Compliment and Positive Self-Talk.

*The minute I heard my first love story,*
*I started looking for you,*
*not knowing how blind that was.*
*Lovers don't finally meet somewhere.*
*They're in each other all along.*

—Rumi

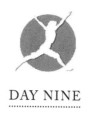

# Love for No Reason–
# Joy for No Reason

What would it feel like to feel Love and Joy for no reason? What if your Being can shine Love and Joy just by *Being*?

Take a minute, close your eyes, and quiet yourself by taking a few slow and deep breaths; feel into Being Love and Being Joy for the sake of Being Love and Being Joy. Nothing to do, nothing to say, just Being in the Glory of Love and Joy.

By adding this to your daily routine, in time, you may find waves of Love and Joy bubbling up inside of you and a soft, perpetual smile on your face.

This is a very powerful practice to do after every meal.

**Being in the question - As you go through your day feel into:**

- ❖ What does it feel like to feel Joy just for the sake of feeling Joy?
- ❖ What does it feel like to feel Happy just for the sake of feeling Happy?
- ❖ What does it feel like to feel Love just for the sake of feeling Love?
- ❖ What does it feel like to be happy to be Alive just for the sake of being Alive?

**Living Words:** Being Love, Being Joy, Being, Nothing to Say and Nothing to Do.

**A Helpful Read:** *Happy for No Reason: 7 Steps to Being Happy from the Inside Out*, by Marci Shimoff, offers you a breakthrough approach to being happy. This book incorporates the latest findings in positive psychology, powerful tools and techniques, moving, real-life stories and a 7-step program that will raise your "happiness set-point."

*No more words.*
*In the name of this place*
*we drink in with our breathing,*
*stay quiet like a flower.*
*So the nightbirds will start singing.*

**—Rumi**

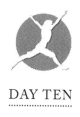

DAY TEN

# Healthy Living–Living Healthy Eating Healthy–Mindful Eating

What if you will feel better and be healthier and possibly live longer and enjoy your life more by eating healthy food, drinking clean water, enjoying each bite (no multitasking – reading, being on the phone or computer, or driving – while eating), blessing your food and being appreciative?

Take time to learn about healthy eating. You will find many helpful resources on the Internet and in the Joyful Living Resources section at the end of this book.

**Food:** The fresher the food you eat, the healthier it is for you, so start a garden in your backyard, join a neighborhood P-Patch (a community vegetable garden where you may grow your own food), learn about sprouts (sprouts are loaded with vitamins, minerals and high in protein), and seek out food that is organic (free of GMOs, pesticides and herbicides). Go Clean! Go Green!

Eat Healthy, sing and send *I Love Yous* to your food as you are preparing your meals. Enjoy your meal with friendly conversation and take pleasure in every bite.

Give thanks for the food before and after each meal.

**Water:** Water is nature's gift to you for better health. Water is vital for helping your body function at its peak, and for eliminating toxins and waste. It is best to drink water that is clear of all chlorine and fluoride. You will find many products on the Internet that will reduce up to 99 percent of chlorine and fluoride from your home's tap water. Clearly Filtered (www.ClearlyFiltered.com) has a full line of top quality water pitchers for your home.

For better health, drinking a glass of warm water with freshly squeezed lemon in the morning will help to clean your kidneys and liver and will wake up your digestive system.

**Extra Credit:** Visualize sparks of light (like a Fourth of July sparkler) going into your water. Sense the sparks of Love, Life and Light as the water rests on your tongue and as it moves into your stomach. See these Divine sparks of Love, Life, Light expanding into and glowing in every cell of your body, illuminating every organ – your kidneys, liver, spleen, heart, lungs, blood, bones, brain, eyes and skin. In time – perhaps weeks, month or years – you may begin to feel the Divine glow of Love, Life and Light from the inside-out.

**Clean Green JUICE:** Get a blender or juicer to juice fruits and veggies every day. Sing *I Love Yous* to the fruits and vegetables as you are preparing them for the juicer. It is best to drink the juice fresh and to not store it. For more info, Google: Juicing.

To improve your overall health, you may choose to reduce your consumption of alcohol to nearly zero, with the exception of a little wine every now and then.

**Being in the question – Take a moment to feel into:**

- ❖ What if one of the finest signs of self-love is lovingly and tenderly taking care of my body?
- ❖ What if eating healthy helps me to feel better, be more mentally clear and emotionally balanced?
- ❖ What if by blessing and saying a prayer of gratefulness over all that I eat and drink, the food and drink will be elevated?
- ❖ What if it is easier to feel joyous and loving when I feel healthy and strong?
- ❖ What would it feel like to be fully Nourished?
- ❖ What would it feel like to have every Cell and every Organ in my body cared for?
- ❖ What would it feel like to be in Glorious Well-being?
- ❖ What would it feel like to give Thanks for all that is given to me?

**Blessing**

Please consider saying a blessing over everything you eat and drink. You may say any prayer that resonates with you or feel free to say the following prayer and visualization.

Blessing the water you drink (or food):

Dear God:
Please Bless this water with Your Divine Love.
Please Bless this water with Your Divine Life.
Please Bless this water with Your Divine Light.
Thank You

**Living Words:** Vigor, Clean, Happy, Healthy, Vibrant, Nourished, Powerful, Magnificent, Strong and Radiant.

# Doctor – Doctor – Doctor

It is much easier to be in Joy when you feel good. Therefore, it is important that you seek out medical support from doctors who you like and trust, such as a medical doctor and a naturopathic doctor to help you strengthen your body. I also recommend that you acquire a life coach or a mentor to help you focus your thinking and balance your emotions.

| | Name | Phone Number |
|---|---|---|
| Doctor: | | |
| Naturopathic Dr.: | | |
| Life Coach/Mentor: | | |
| Chiropractor: | | |
| Masseuse: | | |

What if good health is all about FLOW? To feel great and to be in optimum health, all systems in your body need to flow freely, including your blood, digestion, lymph, energy and emotions. If any of these systems are blocked or restricted by pain or discomfort, disease will develop.

Here are a few self-healing techniques to increase FLOW:

**Back (or other) pain:** Visualize a garden hose that is bent in the middle and not allowing any water to pass through. Now visualize the same garden hose fully unbent with water abundantly flowing. Imagine the bent garden hose where your back pain is located; next, see the hose unbent and fully flowing. Feel the energy flowing in your back. Repeat this for 30 seconds twice a day, and watch to see if the back pain falls away. This technique may be used for pains in all parts of your body.

**Headache:** Use the same garden hose visualization for taming your headaches. Visualize the bent hose in your neck obstructing the flow of water. Next, unbend the hose in your mind and feel the abundant flow of energy. Repeat this for 30–60 seconds, twice a day, as needed.

Peppermint essential oil is a very effective, natural way to lessen your discomfort. Place 10 drops of peppermint oil on a cotton ball, and gently inhale the healing scent. You can also put some peppermint oil in a base oil – (grape-seed oil, sesame-seed oil or olive oil: one part peppermint oil to 10 parts base oil) – and massage the oil onto your temples, forehead, below your nose and on the insides of your wrists. Inhale the oil below your nose, relax and send *I Love Yous* to your headache.

**Healing Pressure Points:** Gently massaging pressure points on your temples, forehead, chest, and on other locations on your body, will help to get energy flowing and reduce your pain. You may learn more by Googling: Acupressure Points.

**Being in the question – Take a moment to feel into:**

- ❖ What does it feel like to be Emotionally Healthy?
- ❖ What does it feel like to be Physically Healthy?
- ❖ What does it feel like to be Mentally Healthy?
- ❖ What does it feel like to be Fully Alive?

**Living Words:** Healthy, Vigor, Aware and Alive.

# Energy Healing

Modern science tells us that everything is energy. Therefore, our bodies, minds and emotions are made up of energy. What if we can improve our health by balancing our energy?

Energy Healing promotes healing by enhancing the flow of energy in your physical body and throughout your energy field or Aura. Greater coherence, flow and balance in the human energy field can facilitate emotional, physical and mental healing.

**Energy Healers:** The following is a list of highly skilled Energy Healers. You will find a vast array of free information and videos on their websites and on YouTube. If this feels good to you, please take the time to learn more about Energy Healing and how it may be beneficial to you. You will find more information in the Joyful Living Resources section.

- ❖ **Panache Desai: www.PanacheDesai.com** – "Stepping Out of Fear and Limitations Experiencing Your Deepest and True Potential"
- ❖ **Julie Renee Doering: www.JulieRenee.com** – "Age Reversal and Master Body Rejuvenator"
- ❖ **Jo Dunning: www.JoDunning.com** – "Discovering the Love You Are"
- ❖ **Matt Kahn: www.TrueDivineNature.com** – "The Love Revolution"
- ❖ **Rikka Zimmerman: www.RikkaZimmerman.com** – "Adventures in Oneness – Awaken to a New World"

**Being in the question – Take a moment to feel into:**

- ❖ What would it feel like to be healthy, vibrant and strong?
- ❖ What would it feel like to be emotionally, physically and mentally in harmony?
- ❖ What if my health will improve by vibrating with the feelings of Joy and Love?
- ❖ What if an Energy Healer can help to guide me towards raising my Joy and Love vibrations?

**Living Words:** Receive, Vibration, Allow, Flow, Harmony, Healthy, Strong and Vibrant.

# Sleep

Your body, mind and spirit will be much happier if every night you have all electronics off by 8:00 p.m., you are in bed by 10:00 p.m., and you are up in the morning by 7:00 a.m. Within a few weeks you may notice that you feel better, you have more energy, your mind is sharper and your emotions are more balanced. Try this for the next 30 days, and each morning write the results in your journal.

**THROW OUT YOUR TV** – However, if you do choose to keep your TV, you may want to limit your viewing to light, entertaining, funny, and educational programs such as *The Cooking Channel, The Travel Channel, Sports, Nature Shows, Dancing with the Stars, The Bachelor* and romantic comedies. Avoid the news, soap operas and talk shows!

**Getting to Sleep** – Here are ideas for helping you to fall asleep:

- ❖ Lavender essential oil on your pillow
- ❖ Warm bath before bed
- ❖ Natural sleep aids from a health-food store—please check with your doctor
- ❖ Filling your mind with happy and loving thoughts
- ❖ Smiling
- ❖ Imagine something you would like to create or invent
- ❖ Counting Sheep – if all else fails

**Being in the question – Take a moment to feel into:**

- ❖ What would it feel like to be fully rested?
- ❖ What would it feel like to take pleasure in my dreams?
- ❖ What would it feel like to be physically strong and mentally awake?

**Living Words:** Rested, Relaxed and Comfortable.

# Breath, Sun and Water

**BREATH:** There is a Life Force in the air you breathe. This Living Energy is called *Chi* in Chinese medicine, in Ayurveda (East Indian medicine) it is called *Prana*, and in the Hebrew Bible it is called *Ruach*. As you go through your day, take slow and deep breaths, be mindful of the vibrant energy that is enlivening every cell in your body, and be grateful. Take walks in nature where the air is cool and fresh.

**SUNSHINE:** All life needs sunlight to live and grow. If you put a plant in a dark room, it will be dead within a few days. Enjoy the sun's Life-Giving Energy. Being in the sunshine naturally lightens your being and puts you in a more joyful mood. The sun helps your body produce Vitamin D. Vitamin D helps to reduce the feelings of depression, so spend time in the sun every day. (Please use common sense and be cautious not to overexpose your skin to sunlight).

**WATER:** Clean, pure water is truly a gift. To increase your health, drink water as you go through your day instead of coffee and beverages that are loaded with sugar.

Swimming in a lake, river or the ocean is one of life's greatest ways to relax, rejuvenate and refresh! A warm salt bath with your favorite essential oils can be like floating in heaven. Spending time in water is a natural and healthy way to bring more Joy, Beauty and Health into your life.

**Living Words:** Breath, Water, Sun, Relax, Rejuvenate, Refresh, Float and Heaven.

*If you want to be more alive,*
*Love is the truest health.*

## —Rumi

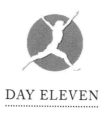

# Anger, Rage, Hate, Guilt, Shame, Sadness

L ife has given us a magnificent array of Emotions!
Life brings us many situations that enliven this magnificent human expression.

So start living and start being fully human. Yes, you have permission to fully express (in a healthy way) your pain, fear, anger, sadness, jealousy, joy, love and power.

## Feel It, Express It, Let It Move through You, and Let It Go

Anger, rage, hate, guilt, shame and sadness are very strong emotions and are a vital part of being human. E-Motion is energy in motion. So feel your anger, your rage, your hate, your guilt, your shame; then express them, embrace their enlivening energy, and finally let them go! We get ourselves stuck (depressed) when we stop our emotions or when we bottle up our feelings and don't allow ourselves to experience our pain, sorrow, loneliness and worry.

**Being in the question – Take a moment to feel into:**

- ❖ What would it feel like to accept my anger as part of me, to welcome it, to celebrate it, to be grateful for it, to send love to it and to let it go?
- ❖ What would it feel like to express my anger in a healthy way?
- ❖ What would it feel like to know that anger is not good or bad?

- What would it feel like to know that anger is part of my life experience?
- What would it feel like to bring more Love and Joy into my life and by doing so, watch anger, rage, hate, guilt, shame and sadness fade from my life?
- What would it feel like to fully express my anger, rage, shame, guilt and sadness?
- What would it feel like to be fully Free of my anger, rage, shame, guilt and sadness?
- What would it feel like to be fully Free?

Below are four powerful exercises that will help you get your locked-up emotions moving out of your cells, organs, body and mind.

1. **I LOVE YOUS**. Send *I Love Yous* to every emotion that arises; send *I Love Yous* to your anger, your rage, your shame and also to your happiness, your accomplishments and your feelings of joy.

2. **Throw a Temper Tantrum.** Yes, get down on all fours and let it rip! Throw a Temper Tantrum just like a three-year-old. Just Do It. A note of caution: You may want to go easy on the Temper Tantrum if you are in the middle of a board meeting at work – some emotions are best expressed in private.

3. **The Tennis Racket Thrust (TRT)** will get your emotions flowing like nothing else. First, put a fluffy feather pillow on a chair. Next, stand in front of the chair with a tennis racket held high above your head with both hands. Then, hit the pillow with your full strength while you thrust your pelvis forward, saying loudly: "I Love You!" Continue this with full strength for one to three minutes. Make sure to time yourself. Again, you may want to do this exercise when no one else is around. Do this every day and watch your anger fade away.
By saying "I Love You," you are sending a reset message to your mind and emotions. The goal here is to express and clear out your anger. There is no guarantee that you will come to love

the person or situation with whom/which you are angry after completing this exercise, though it is exhilarating when that happens, too.

4. Take a kickboxing class or try any contact activity.

**Living Words:** Express, Release, Flow, Power and Free.

*This being human is a guest house.*
*Every morning a new arrival.*

*A joy, a depression, a meanness,*
*some momentary awareness comes*
*as an unexpected visitor.*

*Welcome and entertain them all!*
*. . . treat each guest honorably. . .*

*The dark thought, the shame, the malice.*
*Meet them at the door laughing and*
*invite them in.*

*Be grateful for whatever comes*
*because each has been sent*
*as a guide from beyond.*

—Rumi

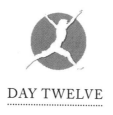

DAY TWELVE

# Forgiveness – Letting Go

*Forgiving Others and Forgiving Myself*

Here you are on Day 12. Take a deep breath, smile and pat yourself on the back – you have worked (played) hard and you can feel grateful for your progress.

For many people, forgiveness is all but impossible; it is like standing on the highest mountain and not seeing a path to the valley. The emotions of anger, guilt, shame and rage can be all too powerful and can feel impossible to wade through. Yet, to find real joy and peace, one must find a way into forgiveness.

## Ho'oponopono

Here is a Magic Carpet that will help you fly over your mountain of emotions and bring you safely into the valley of peace. *Ho'oponopono* (the *o* is pronounced with a long "ooo") is a mystical Hawaiian chant that works on physical, mental, emotional and spiritual levels to clear a person's anger, guilt, shame and rage, allowing complete forgiveness to begin.

*Ho'oponopono* consists of four powerful lines and is very easy to commit to memory. It may be spoken out loud to the person you want to forgive, or you may speak it to yourself with the person in mind. It's also very powerful for forgiving oneself. We have all made mistakes in this life and we can forgive ourselves by recalling the mistake and speaking the four lines with conviction.

*I am sorry*
*Please forgive me*
*Thank you*
*I love you*

*Ho'oponopono* has a cumulative effect, so say it often and say it with feeling!

Check out this You Tube video to learn more: **www.thereisaway. org/Ho'oponopono_cleaning_meditation.htm**.

Here is a touching story that speaks to the very depth of Forgiveness: During the many years of apartheid in South Africa, some of humanity's worst atrocities occurred. When the apartheid government fell, a program of Reconciliation was created to help heal the country. For a person to be free from being convicted for the crimes that he or she had committed, that person had to face the individual who suffered the act. In one such case, a young white soldier who had killed a black man had to face the dead man's widow. When the widow saw the man who had killed her husband, she said, "I forgive you completely, and I have three demands: First, I want us to go to the location where my husband was killed and burned to collect some of the soil containing his ashes, so that I can give my husband a burial with that soil. Second, I want to adopt you as my son, since we had no children, so that I can love you as the child we never had. Third, I want you to come and visit me once a month." She went on to say, "And to show you that I fully forgive you, I will give you a hug." As she walked over to the soldier, all the people in the courtroom started to sing "Amazing Grace," and the solder fainted.

Life brings us many joys and Life brings us challenges and pain. The goal here is to experience all of it, then let it go and return to Love.

True Forgiveness will set you free – Just Let Go . . .

**Being in the question – Take a moment to feel into:**

- ❖ What would it feel like to fully Forgive Everyone?
- ❖ What would it feel like to fully Forgive Life?
- ❖ What would it feel like to Completely Forgive Myself?

**Living Words:** Release, Harmony, Peace, Forgiven and Forgiving.

*The wound is the place where
the Light enters you.*

## —Rumi

*Goodbyes are only for those who love with
their eyes. Because for those who love with
heart and soul, there is no such thing as
separation.*

## —Rumi

*A thousand half-loves must be forsaken to
take one whole heart home.*

## —Rumi

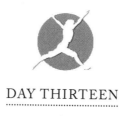

# Making Friends With God

## *Divine Allowing – Allowing the Divine*

A friend is one who Loves you, Supports you, and who is there for you through the good times and the not-so-good times.

What if God is that friend? What if God loves you more than you know? It is said that the moment you were born, God, the Creator of the Universe, had His full attention on you!

What if Being in the Grace of God is all that is essential?

You are a magnificent creation of the Creator of the Universe. You are truly loved. Feel that Love!

You are a child of God. It is natural for every parent to want his or her child to be Happy, Healthy and Prosperous!

The best way to feel God's Love is to give God your love and your gratitude, to love and appreciate His Creation and to be joyful.

> *You are an Eternal Expression of the Divine –*
> *What a joy it is to walk this earth knowing who*
> *you are and shining the Love, Joy and Grace of*
> *God in all that you say, think and do!*

**Being in the question – Take a moment to feel into:**

- ❖ What would it feel like to wake up every morning feeling, *Thank God I Am Alive!*?
- ❖ What would it feel like to fully give my love to God?
- ❖ What would it feel like to completely Trust God?
- ❖ What would it feel like to be safe in the Grace of God?

- What would it feel like to be fully comforted in the Love of God?
- What would it feel like to truly appreciate all the gifts God has given me?
- What would it feel like to know that God loves me?
- What would it feel like to radiate full abundance from God?
- What would it feel like to know that there is a Divine Plan for all Life?
- What would it feel like to joyfully surrender to the Divine Plan for my Life?
- What would it feel like to know Divine Safety, Support, Joy, Mastery, Confidence and Peace?

# Bringing God into Your Life
# Through Love and Prayer

A beautiful way to bring God into your life is to bring more Love into your life and into the lives of others; to be an emissary of God's Love in this world.

Heartfelt prayers are powerful. The best way to create a friendship is to talk to God. Here are some suggested prayers:

## Morning: Before Rising

*This is the day that the Lord hath made;*
*I will rejoice and be glad in it.*

– Psalm 118:24, King James Bible

*Dear God, the Creator of the Universe, You are full of mercy and compassion. Thank you for returning my soul to me. May I bring Your Love, Light, Joy and Wisdom into the world this day.*

Before each meal, pause to reflect on the Source of the food you are about to eat. Bless the food and be grateful to God for creating that which you are about to eat.

## A prayer for your day:

*I Am in the Love of God.*
*I Am in the Light of God.*
*I Am in the Life of God.*
*I Am in the Beauty of God.*
*I Am in the Grace of God.*
*I Am in the Abundance of God.*

*I Shine the Love of God into all Life.*
*I Shine the Light of God into all Life.*
*I Shine the Life of God into all Life.*
*I Shine the Beauty of God into all Life.*
*I Shine the Grace of God into all Life.*
*I Shine the Abundance of God into all Life.*

*Thank You, God.*
*Thank You, God.*
*Thank You, God.*

## Before going to sleep:

Reflect on your day and give thanks to God for all the gifts that you have received. Send God your love and gratitude. Also send love and gratitude to your body, being mindful of all that it has done for you – from digesting to seeing, from walking to talking, from feeling to loving.

You may want to add the following to your morning meditation or to your nightly prayers:

*I Allow Divine Love to Fill My Entire Being.*
*I Allow Myself to Fully Love Myself.*
*I Allow for Divine Healing in My Life.*
*I Allow for Divine Grace to Enlighten Me.*
*I Allow for Divine Abundance in Every Part of My Life.*
*I Allow for the Divine to Fill Me with Divine Wisdom.*
*I Allow for the Divine to Fill Me with Complete Faith.*
*I Allow for the Divine to Fill Me with Pure Peace.*

**A prayer for gaining Divine Guidance** (This prayer may be repeated many times during your day):

*Dear Holy God,*
*Here I am.*
*I am ready.*
*I am open.*
*Guide me.*
*Thank You, God*
*I Love You, God.*

**Living Words:** Love, Loved, Gratitude, Grace, Friendship, Wisdom, Centered, Balance, Connected, Blessed, Mastery, Confidence, Peace, Abundance, Radiance, Harmony and Joy.

**A Helpful Read:**

*Conversations With God*, by Neale Donald Walsch, **www.CWG. org**, is a best selling book, with over seven million copies sold. This book is easy to read and offers you great insights to some of life's most profound questions such as the nature of God, love, faith, life, death, good and discovering your life's purpose.

*I am so close, I may look distant.*
*So completely mixed with you,*
*I may look separate.*
*So out in the open, I appear hidden.*
*So silent, because I am constantly*
*talking with you.*

—Rumi

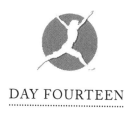

# Meditation

*Inner Peace – Inner Wisdom – Inner Knowing*

Medical research has shown proof of the many physical and emotional benefits a person receives from engaging in a regular meditation practice. Some of the benefits include lowering blood pressure, helping to heal depression and gaining more joy, clarity, patience and a sense of fulfillment in life.

Meditation is easy to learn and by adding 10–20 minutes of meditation in the morning and evening to your daily schedule, you will soon feel more peaceful in life.

## The Power Of Meditation

*The Power Of Large Groups Meditating Together –*
*Creating A More Peaceful World*

Much scientific research has been done showing that when a large group of people come together to meditate – (via Transcendental Meditation) – they have a positive effect on the entire location; and the larger the group, the more profound the results.

For decades, the nations of Egypt and Israel have fought horrific battles with each other. In 1978, both nations declared that they were tired of war; and with the help of then United States President, Jimmy Carter, the presidents of Egypt and Israel met with the goal of establishing peace. Sadly, however, late in 1978, the talks between the two leaders dissipated, with no expectation of the talks resuming.

With the goal of reviving the peace talks and ultimately of creating a more coherent atmosphere in the Middle East, Maharishi Mahesh Yogi, the founder of Transcendental Meditation, asked TM mediators from the US to travel to the city of Safed in Northern Israel for the cause. I enthusiastically joined with over 500 of my fellow meditators on this mission for peace. For two and a half months, we spent long hours in the mornings and afternoons practicing an advanced technique called the TM Sidhis Program. The goal was to help create an atmosphere to facilitate the leaders of Egypt and Israel to revisit their peace talks and to complete a peace agreement. Within one month of our presence in Israel, the talks were back on, and within two months, the leaders of both countries sat down to initial the completed peace agreement.

Right now may be a perfect time for us all to practice meditation daily for our personal wellbeing and for the wellbeing of all life on earth.

Transcendental Meditation is easy to learn and is one of the most popular and effective forms of meditation. There are Transcendental Meditation centers in most major cities around the world. To locate a center near you go to: **www.TM.org**.

## Being Still – The Power of Stillness

*Being* is the home of the Unified Field of All Possibilities that give rise to all Life. *Being* is the home of all Pure Love, Power, Beauty, Truth, Knowledge, Abundance, Joy and Wisdom. So Be in *Being*!

### *Being* is silence in motion

Take 10 minutes right now sitting in silence with your eyes closed (be comfortable and ensure that you are not disturbed). Take three deep and slow breaths, completely relax, close your eyes, and then slowing breathe into the feelings of:

❖ What would it feel like to Be Love?
  **Be Love** for a full minute

❖ What would it feel like to Be Power?
  **Be Power** for a full minute.

❖ What would it feel like to Be Beauty?
  **Be Beauty** for a full minute.

❖ What would it feel like to Be Truth?
  **Be Truth** for a full minute.

❖ What would it feel like to Be Knowledge?
  **Be Knowledge** for a full minute.

❖ What would it feel like to Be Abundance?
  **Be Abundance** for a full minute.

❖ What would it feel like to Be Joy?
  **Be Joy** for a full minute.

❖ What would it feel like to Be Wisdom?
  **Be Wisdom** for a full minute.

❖ What would it feel like to Be Still?
  **Be Still** for a full minute.

What if by spending 10 minutes twice a day – (once in the morning and once before you go to sleep) – in the silent *Being* of Love, Power, Beauty, Truth, Knowledge, Abundance, Joy and Wisdom, in time, this *Being* of Love, Power, Beauty, Truth, Knowledge, Abundance, Joy and Wisdom will become YOU?

The following is a very powerful stillness meditation:

*Be Still And Know That I Am God*
*Be Still And Know That I Am*
*Be Still And Know*
*Be Still*
*Be*

**Being in the question – Take a moment to feel into:**

- ❖ What would it feel like to Be?
- ❖ What would it feel like to Be in Transcendence?
- ❖ What would it feel like to Be in Peace?
- ❖ What would it feel like to Be Connected with My Higher Self?
- ❖ What would it feel like to Be Connected with My Higher Knowing?

**Living Words:** Being, Breath, Brilliant, Centered, Silence, Peace, Quiet, All Knowing, Transcend and Complete.

*Each moment contains a hundred messages from God.*

## —Rumi

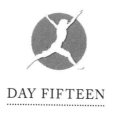

# Beauty

### *Beauty Is Joy in Form*

What if the more Beauty you experience, the more you will naturally be in Joy?

What would it feel like to bring Beauty into all that you say and everything you do?

What would it feel like to be the artist of your life?

What would it feel like to create a beautiful home, inside and out, a beautiful marriage, children, community and a beautiful Life?

From this moment forward, look for ways to bring Beauty into your Life. Look to filling every moment with Beauty. With every breath you take, with every step you make, add beauty to your life and to all life on earth.

Add beauty to the way you walk, to the way you talk, to the way you dress, to the way you design your bedroom, living room, kitchen, bathroom and office.

**Make beauty your essence** so that your *Being* is shining with beauty at all times, in every situation and in every relationship.

Bringing Beauty into your life can be as simple as putting fresh flowers on the dining room table, cleaning out a closet, writing a beautiful poem, feeling how beautiful you are as you look in a mirror, or lifting a friend's spirits by telling her/him that she/he is beautiful.

Here are four ways that I am going to bring more Beauty into my Life:

1. _____

_____

2. _____

_____

3. _____

_____

4. _____

_____

**Being in the question – Take a moment to feel into:**

- ❖ What would it feel like to fully Express My Inner Beauty?
- ❖ What would it feel like to enjoy all the Beauty around Me?
- ❖ What would it feel like to Create Beauty?

**Living Words:** Beauty, Creation, Brilliance, Love and Joy.

*I see my beauty in you.*

—Rumi

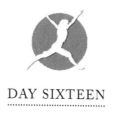

# Adventure

*Make Your Life an Adventure!*
*Explore, Learn, Expand Your Wisdom, Enjoy the Wonder!*

Travel through life, living and looking with the eyes of a three-year-old – being caught up in the mystery, wonder and excitement of this beautiful adventure we call life.

**Explore:** Plan a getaway every month. It can be a trip to a museum, a sporting event, the theater or just spending a day with friends you have not seen in years. The getaway can be more extensive, of course, such as a three-day weekend to a spa, a national park or a workshop.

**Travel:** Once every year, plan a major exploration: Spend two weeks in the Swiss Alps, Jerusalem, Bali, Argentina, the pyramids of Egypt or Italy – yes, Italy!

**Learn:** Become an expert. Choose a subject that you have a high interest in and become a master in that field. It can be anything that gets you excited such as children, sex, marriage, astrology, astronomy, essential oils, health, the body, how the eyes work, Texas, George Washington, Van Gogh or politics. Every year choose a new topic to master. Have fun!

**Wisdom:** Gain Wisdom. Wisdom is inner knowledge that will help you discern correct thought and action—bringing happiness and success to your life and shining joy to your heart and soul. Wisdom is cultivated from quiet reflection, from deep meditation, from reading inspiring books, from associating with people who possess great wisdom, and from learning from life's experiences.

**Italy: The Great Adventure** – Fun, Beauty, Diamonds, Intrigue, Romance and Danger.

Some years ago, I had the honor of dating a very special girl, Angelina, (not her real name), who happened to be a gemologist for a high-end jewelry store in Seattle. One day her client, Michael, (not his real name), walked into the store and asked Angelina to design and create a diamond bracelet with 35 individual ¾ karat diamonds plus a 1¼ karat flawless diamond in the middle. Michael's romantic plan was to have the diamond bracelet delivered to him in Positano, Italy, where he would lovingly propose to his girlfriend. The diamond bracelet would be a small token of his love.

Angelina designed the piece and the store had it made. There was one small problem: Figuring out how to deliver the diamond dazzler to Michael in Italy. A courier would be too expensive, and shipping it to a hotel in Italy would be too risky. The solution: Angelina would fly to Positano and personally deliver the bracelet. Being the gentleman that I am, I stepped forward to be her bodyguard on this adventure. And what an adventure it turned out to be!

With the jewels safely strapped to Angelina in a body belt, we took flight – from Seattle, to Copenhagen, to Rome, then finally to our destination in Naples.

Upon landing in Naples, we went directly to the rental car agency where we met Lorenzo, (Possibly his real name), a young 18-year-old Italian man who was hanging out flirting with his girlfriend, the manager of the agency. We hired Lorenzo to drive us the two hours down the coast to Michael's hotel in Positano. Naples drivers drive like they are in competition for an Olympic gold medal, and we needed a native competitor!

We set off dodging cars through the narrow streets of Naples, winding down and around the most majestic coastline—the shimmering Mediterranean Sea.

Angelina and I were blissfully enjoying the warm Italian air and the beauty unfolding around us as we made our way along the Almalfi coast to Positano.

We arrived at Michael's hotel two minutes before our prearranged time to meet. We had just flown halfway around the world, and we arrived 120 seconds early. Right as Angelina and I stepped into the hotel, we saw Michael walking into the lobby– what perfect timing!

The three of us walked out of the hotel and down an old stone walkway to a private beach on the Mediterranean Sea. We sat at a round table with great anticipation. Angelina laid out the diamond bracelet. We sat there, in the warm Italian sun, with the glistening sea in front of us and the ancient cliffs of the Amalfi coast standing majestically behind. How could it get any better? Michael was wowed by the diamonds, and as he was about to sign off on receiving the jewels, Lorenzo came running down the stairs; the last bus to Naples was about to leave and I had not paid him for his chauffeuring services. When Lorenzo saw the diamond bracelet, his eyes got bigger than two peaches. I quickly pulled him to the side, gave him the twenty dollars I had promised him, and ushered him up the stairs. I can imagine the stories he told his girlfriend when he got back to Naples!

Michael treated Angelina and myself to dinner that night at the 5-star hotel – and what a dinner it was! Michael was set to propose to his girlfriend (with the diamond bracelet) that night at dinner. We sat outside on the beautiful dining patio watching the sun setting on the Mediterranean – with lush grape vines hanging above us, and a glowing fire cooking our fish and pasta just a few feet away. On the romantic scale, this felt like a TEN.

Michael asked us not to make eye contact when he proposed– but how could we not at least watch? As he opened the case to show the bracelet to his soon-to-be-fiancé, I could see the brilliant colors of the diamonds as they danced in the fire-light.

His fiancé's smile spread from cheek to cheek as she said *Yes!*

A few minutes later Michael came over to our table and introduced us to his fiance'. Love *and* Italy – how could life get any better? And that was just the beginning of our week-long adventure in one of the most romantic locations in the world!

Angelina and I woke early the following morning and jumped on the hydrofoil that took us to the island of Capri and the Blue Grotto. When we arrived on Capri, I hired a driver, Mario, (possibly his real name), to tour us around in his convertible. For the next 8 hours, Mario showed us the sights, sounds and character of the island, from private little beaches, to cozy cafés, to the Blue Grotto.

The next day we headed to the romantic little town of Amalfi where I hired Peppi, (not his real name), with horse and carriage. Peppi had to be in his eighties and spoke only Italian. His horse was named Trigger. Trigger boasted a four-foot-high white plume on his head, and performed tricks for our amusement. As we settled into the carriage, Peppi placed a blanket over our legs; then – with the snap of the whip – we rode off into our own little romantic paradise. Construction workers yelled, "*Bella, Bella, Muta Bella!*" *(Beautiful, Beautiful, Very Beautiful!)* from atop their scaffoldings, as we weaved slowly through Amalfi's charming, narrow streets. They weren't bellowing that to me. If they had roses, they surely would have showered Angelina with them. We loved every minute of our Italian adventure.

I will leave the rest of our story to your imagination.

Next time someone offers you the opportunity for a new adventure, you may want to jump in – especially if it involves Italy.

Here are my next four adventures:

1. _____

2. _____

3. _____

4. _____

**Being in the question – Take a moment to feel into:**

- ❖ What would it feel like to fully enjoy Life's Adventure?
- ❖ What would it feel like to be in the delight of Wonder?
- ❖ What would it feel like to be on the Beach in Hawaii with My Lover?
- ❖ What would it feel like to Create a Life of Adventure?

**Living Words:** Adventure, Wisdom, Explore, Grow, Expand, Learn, Quest, Perceive and Italy.

*Travel brings power and love*
*back into your life.*

—Rumi

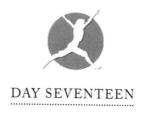

# Abundance

*Change Your Seed Thought – Change Your Life*

**A**bundance – Yes, life is much more fun when you are living in the abundance of money, health and love. There is a joy that comes from living in a comfortable home, traveling the world in style, paying for your children's college educations, and knowing that you have more than enough money to retire in comfort.

What if your inner programming (your seed thought) is keeping you from swimming in abundance?

What if you have the ability to reprogram your seed thought and, in so doing, you begin to live in greater abundance?

What if more abundance will naturally flow into your life when you move your seed thought from lack, self-pity and feelings of *not good enough,* to healthier seed thoughts of Capable, Commanding, Certain, Happy, Wealthy and Confident?

**Seed Thought:**

A seed thought is your inner self (your subconscious) talking to you. It is like a computer program that is running 24/7 telling you who you are (your self-talk). If your seed thought is: "I like myself, I am happy, I am successful, I am abundant, I am magnificent," then it is very likely that you will like yourself, be happy, be successful, be abundant and be magnificent! If your seed thought is: "I am poor, I am sad, I am fat, I am sick," it is very likely that you will be poor, sad, fat and sick!

**Changing Your Seed Thought:**

What if you can create a more positive seed thought by sending *I Love Yous* to everything that life brings you? What if every *I Love You* that you send to a negative thought helps to lessen its power, and in time, change it to a more positive thought?

**Five Ways to Change Your Seed Thought from Negative to Positive:**

1. Send *I Love Yous* to every thought, both positive and negative.

2. As you go through your day, feel into the power of Living Words such as Happy, Brilliant, Healthy, Wealthy, Fun, Joy, Love, Powerful, Certain and Capable. As you walk through your day, make these words the foundation of who you are, so that your essences is Happy, Brilliant, Healthy, Wealthy, Fun, Joy, Love, Powerful, Certain and Capable.

3. Daily silent meditation will help you to clean out your negative seed thoughts and give you a greater sense of well-being. You may also want to bring into your daily routine a guided meditation such as *Abundance Waterfall* and *Liquid Luck*, by Joseph Gallenberger. These guided meditations are very powerful and may help you to move into more Joy and Abundance: **www.synccreation.com**.

4. Seek to spend time with people who are happy and successful.

5. Have fun! Play! Dream! Relax! Make your life a fun adventure!

**Money Loves Excitement:**

If you would like to see more money come into your life, getting excited just might be the key!

First thing in the morning, as you jump out of bed, DECLARE WITH A HAPPY CONFIDENCE: *"I am excited about all the joy, adventure and money that is coming into my life today!"* Then, let it go while keeping a spark of this excitement in your heart and in your smile as you go through your day; and with GRATITUDE, watch what life brings you.

**Fake It until You Make It:**

If you are having trouble feeling excited, you may need to fake it until you make it. Keep at it. In time, your mornings will start with a new sense of excitement, enthusiasm and joy... and an expanded bank account.

**Money Loves:**

Money Loves Confidence, Trust, Generosity, Graciousness, Honesty, Fairness, A well-thought-out Business Plan, Energy, Action, Saving 10 percent and Giving 10 percent towards making life better for others.

**Three Steps to Creating Wealth:**

1. Create a financial plan where your income is greater than your expenses. Week by week, take the actions necessary to implement your financial plan. As you go through your day, look for opportunities that will increase your income and reduce your expenses. Feel the power and confidence that comes from putting together your financial plan and from boldly taking the steps to put it into action.

2. Start saving today. Every month put a specific amount of dollars (perhaps 5–10 percent of your income) into savings and watch your wealth grow. There is a pleasant and secure feeling that comes with knowing that you have money set aside for emergencies, vacations, retirement and savings.

3. Be a happy Tither. Every month, with a happy heart and a smile on your face give 10 percent (or a set amount that is comfortable for you) of your income to help make someone else's life better. There seems to be a Universal Law that states that the more you give, the more will be given to you.

Who is wealthy? One who is appreciative of all that they have. Are you Wealthy? You can be, right now.

**Being in the question – Take a moment to feel into:**

- ❖ What would it feel little to have over-flowing Abundance in all areas of my life including Health, Wealth, Work, Family and Friends?
- ❖ What would it feel like to have my self-talk be fill with I am Capable, Commanding, Certain, Happy, Wealthy, Healthy and Confident?
- ❖ What would it feel like to be a Joyful Receiver and a Happy Giver?

**Helpful Reads:**

*Financial Peace University* by Dave Ramsey, **www.DaveRamsey. com**. Dave Ramsey offers you a complete financial plan for getting your finances in order, from getting out of debt to building a large money reserve that will help you have an elevated peace of mind about your finances.

*Think and Grow Rich* by Napoleon Hill. This book will offer you new thoughts and ideas that will help you to create greater success.

*Yes to Success!* By Debra Poneman, **www.YesToSuccess.com**. Debra has been guiding and inspiring people to live more successful and happier lives for over 30 years.

**Living Words:** Wealthy, Income, Cash Flow, Saving, Giving, Energy, Excited, Content, Thankful, Happy, Brilliant, Healthy, Fun, Joy, Love, Powerful, Certain and Capable.

*Let yourself be silently drawn by*
*the strange pull of what you really love.*
*It will not lead you astray.*

### —Rumi

DAY EIGHTEEN

# Fun

**M**erriam-Webster's defines *fun* as, "what provides amusement or enjoyment; *specifically*: playful, often boisterous action or speech."

The real definition of fun is: that which brings a Smile to your face and Joy to your Heart!

**Your Daily Fun Requirement**

Put some fun in your life every day! The more fun you have, the more you will experience joyfulness, 24/7... even to the point of smiling in your sleep!

Take time right now to write down six activities that will bring a Smile to your face and Joy to your Heart. Here are a few ideas:

1. Playing with children
2. Dancing Swing, Polka, Waltz, Blues, Salsa
3. A friendly/competitive game of tennis or any sport
4. Romantic play
5. Travel
6. Gardening
7. Professional Roller Derby
8. Playing in water: swimming, sailing, paddle boarding, river kayaking, water polo
9. Exploring . . .

**The following are six fun activities that I will bring into my life:**

1. _____

_____

2. _____

_____

3. _____

_____

4. _____

_____

5. _____

_____

6. _____

_____

**Being in the question – Take a moment to feel into:**

❖ What would it feel like to be rolling on the floor laughing with a three-year-old?

❖ What would it feel like to play an exhilarating game of tennis?

❖ What would it feel like to be swept off your feet on the dance floor?

❖ What would it feel like to experience all of life with a happy heart?

**Living Words:** Fun, Laugh, Dance, Joy, Happy, Exhilaration and Adventure.

*I drank water from your spring
and felt the current take me.*

—Rumi

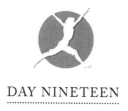

# Romance

Are you ready for some sensuous fun? Romance, Sensuality and Love are some of the greatest joys in life and *now* is your time to enliven more spice and sparkle! Are you ready?

**Massage: Fun, Healthy and Sexy…**
A good massage will relax the body, refresh the mind and sooth your soul.

Have your partner massage your body from head to toe in the morning before you even get out of bed. Have your lover send *I Love Yous* to every part of your body as he/she is warmly and tenderly massaging you. Choose your favorite scented oils and make this intimate time fun, sexy and playful. Tell your partner that these are "Doctor's Orders." **Make sure you reward your partner for the pleasure he/she is giving you and make it fun for the both of you.**

You may want to seek out a professional masseuse if you do not have a partner. As you receive your massage, enjoy the loving feelings and thoughts that arise, and revel in your sensuality.

You are a passionate and sensual person—Live it, Love it, Scream it!

**The Sensuous Woman – Wear sexy lingerie all the time.** Yes, you have full permission to be Loving, Sensuous and Sexy. If you like, you may wear silky underwear to bed, to work, while cooking, when you are out dancing or at a party. Feel your sexuality; revel in your Femininity. There is Great Power and Joy to be expressed and experienced in the full display of your natural sensuality – (please do use some discretion when in public). If you are in a relationship, you may want to reserve the joys of your sensuality for the love in your life.

**The Sensuous Man – Wear Chivalry, Generous Confidence and Masculinity 24/7.** A man stands in his Masculinity when he expresses his nobility, courage, honor, loyalty and thoughtfulness towards the woman in his life. So feel into your power, your wisdom and your softness, as these qualities will arouse strength in you and kindle passion in your lover.

**Single?** Are you single and ready to be with the Love of your Life? What if you can call on the loving power of the Universe to bring your life partner to you by raising your level of joy combined with heartfelt intension?

**A Helpful Read:** *Calling In The One,* by Katherine Woodward Thomas, **wwwKatherineWoodwardThomas.com**.

**Married?** Are you ready to enliven a deeper Love, a Joyful Sparkle and more Richness with your partner? If you are, here is a recipe: Combine 8 cups of Self-Love, 6 cups of Forgiveness, 4 cups of shared mission and goals, creativity and no expectations, 2 cups of romance, sensuality, vulnerability, playfulness and laughter, 1 cup of financial abundance, adventure, weekend getaways and charm. Heat at 360 degrees with a tender, generous, grateful and loving heart, for the rest of your life.

**A Helpful Read:** *The Soulmate Secret: Three Keys To Manifesting True Love,* by Arielle Ford, **www.ArielleFord.com**.

Katherine Woodward Thomas and Arielle Ford are two world-renowned relationship professionals who offer great insights and tools to assist you in attracting and deepening true and lasting love relationships.

**Here are four ways that I am bringing more Love, Sensuality and Playfulness into my life:**

1. _____

_____

2. _____

_____

3. _____

_____

4. _____

_____

**Being in the question – Take a moment to feel into:**

- ❖ What does it feel like to Love my body?
- ❖ What does it feel like to feel attractive?
- ❖ What does it feel like to relax into my pleasure?
- ❖ What does it feel like to be abundantly Sexy?
- ❖ What does it feel like to Express My Sensuality?
- ❖ What does it feel like to fully Surrender into my Femininity and Stand in my Masculinity? (Everyone is part feminine and part masculine).

**Living Words:** Excited, Soft, Vulnerable, Nobility, Love, Warmth, Erotic, Sensuous, Luxurious and Power.

*That which God said to the rose,*
*and caused it to laugh in full-blown beauty,*
*He said to my heart,*
*and made it a hundred times more beautiful.*

—Rumi

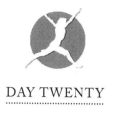

# Take This Day Off

## *Relax and Enjoy*

Take this day off. You have been working/playing very diligently. You deserve a day all to yourself.

Make this a time to relax and enjoy yourself. You may want to take long baths and beautiful walks, share time with family and friends or relish in this time devoted just to yourself.

This is your day to En-Joy!

### Sabbath – A Day Apart To Recharge, Unwind And Unplug.

What would it feel like to devote one day a month or one day a week, perhaps a Saturday or Sunday, to spending time with family and friends, relaxing, enjoying a two hour lunch, relishing in personal and spiritual growth, taking a hike or just hanging out reading a good book?

What would it feel like to have a day completely void of distractions from things such as your TV, computer and, yes, even your phone?

You may call this day whatever you choose: a Sabbath, an island in time, "my time to recharge," or "my day of joy."

The goal here is to set a specific time to relax your body, mind, emotions and soul. Taking this time for yourself will enable you to function at a higher level, receive inspiration and enjoy life more fully.

**Being in the question – Take a moment to feel into:**

- ❖ What would it feel like to have one day a week set aside for me to rest and recharge?
- ❖ What would it feel like to have time all to myself?
- ❖ What would it feel like to fully relax?
- ❖ What would it feel like to fully enjoy?
- ❖ What would it feel like to Be...?

**Living Words:** Sabbath, time all to myself, relaxed, refreshed, unplugged and recharged.

*We often need to be refreshed.*

## —Rumi

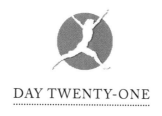

# Gratitude

What if **Heartfelt Gratitude** is a fundamental ingredient necessary for feeling the full richness of Joy?

What if your life will be lifted to new heights by giving **Heartfelt Gratitude** to every experience life brings you?

Scientific research has shown that people who feel and express Gratitude are happier, healthier, live longer and are wealthier than people who lack Gratitude in their lives.

Therefore a key to a happier, healthier, longer and more abundant life is **Heartfelt Gratitude**.

**Giving Gratitude:** There is something very special about this miracle we call Life. The fact that you are alive – your heart is beating, your body is breathing and your eyes are reading this – is a miracle beyond wonder! As you go through your day, take pause and feel deep **Heartfelt Gratitude** for all the miracles that come to you every second.

**Receiving Gratitude:** Pause for a moment when someone thanks you or sends you a word of praise. Breathe in each compliment, for it is a gift of life shining a drop of Joy to your Being.

**Take The Gratitude Challenge For The Next Thirty Days:** Each day find at least 10 things for which you are entirely Grateful. Each night, lovingly record all of your "Gratitudes" from the day in your journal. After the thirty days, notice whether you are feeling happier, healthier and even wealthier.

Now make expressing **Heartfelt Gratitude** a fundamental part of your daily life.

**Here is what I am Grateful for:**

1. _____
_____

2. _____
_____

3. _____
_____

4. _____
_____

5. _____
_____

6. _____
_____

7. _____
_____

8. _____
_____

9. _____
_____

10. _____
_____

**Being in the question – Take a moment to feel into:**

- ❖ What would it feel like to be fully Grateful for my life?
- ❖ What would it feel like to be fully Humble?
- ❖ What would it feel like to fully relax into Graciousness?
- ❖ What would it feel like to value all that life brings me?
- ❖ What would it feel like to lovingly receive a compliment?

**Living Words:** Gratitude, Joy, Peace, Grateful, Praise, Wealth, Health, Long and Happy Life and Thank You God!

*Thankfulness brings you to the place where the Beloved lives.*

## —Rumi

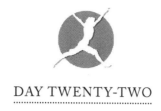

DAY TWENTY-TWO

# Loving What Arises

What if your life is an exciting adventure ride, full of "ups" and "downs?" What if this adventurous ride you are on will be much more enjoyable by *Loving What Arises*? Yes, loving everything: The pains and the joys, the loves and the heartaches, the peace and the stress.

Today, and for the rest of your life, bring into your being the rewarding feeling of Loving all that comes your way, and watch as life brings you more delight and less darkness. Any darkness that does arise will lose some of its charge.

The secret here is to boldly move your life forward, holding a clear vision of the life of your dreams, as you send *Love to All That Arises*.

If you are in a toxic or abusive relationship, a change may be necessary. Please seek appropriate counseling.

**Being in the question – Take a moment to feel into:**

❖ What if by Loving everything life brings me, my life will flow with more grace and ease?

❖ What if by lovingly asking of all that life brings me, "What else is possible?" the Universe will give me new and more joyful adventures?

**Living Words:** Love, Joy, Flow, Grace, Ease, Boldness and Vision.

**A Helpful Read:**
*Whatever Arises, Love That: A Love Revolution That Begins With You*, by Matt Kahn, **www.TrueDivineNature.com**. Matt Kahn is a vibration healer who offers you meaningful insights that will add

charm to your life. In his new book, he richly explores ways to help you bring your highest self forward in all that life brings you.

*Yesterday I was clever,*
*so I wanted to change the world.*
*Today I am wise,*
*so I am changing myself.*

## —Rumi

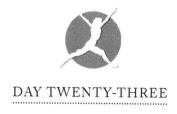

..............................................................

# Create

S how the world your unique talents and gifts by creating something magnificent such as: A painting, a poem, a book, a delicious meal, an educational website, a happy and abundant life, techniques to help others live a happy and abundant life, a dress, a home, a ceramic vase, a program for meaningful social change, a baby!

Have fun while you are exploring your creative talents to make something. There is a great joy that you will naturally feel when you create something new and exciting.

**Creating A Better World:** Look to create that which will bring more Beauty and Joy into the world. Bring out your highest creativity to make the world more Joyful, Peaceful and Beautiful place for you, your family, your community and for future generations.

**This Week and in the Weeks Ahead I Will Create:**

1. _____

    _____

2. _____

    _____

3. _____

    _____

4. _____

_____

5. _____

_____

6. _____

_____

**Being in the question – Take a moment to feel into:**

- ❖ What would it feel like to let my creative talents flow?
- ❖ What would it feel like to create something Beautiful?
- ❖ What would it feel like to be acknowledged and honored for my talents?
- ❖ What would it feel like to help create a better world?

**Living Words:** Talent, Creation, Creativity, Beauty, Fun and Honored.

*Do not be satisfied with the stories
that come before you.
Unfold your own myth.*

## —Rumi

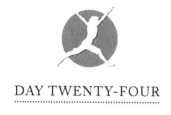

# Living a Meaningful Life

The formula for living a meaningful life can be easy, fun and enlivening!

Are you ready? Here we go!

1. **Be Love**. Giving Love and receiving Love is the essence of who you are, for Love will open doors in miraculous ways.

2. **Go Forth Shining Your Brilliance**, for your Brilliance is a God-given gift that this world desperately needs. As you shine, you will inspire others to do the same.

> *Don't ask what the world needs. Ask what makes*
> *you come alive, and go and do it. Because what*
> *the world needs is people who have come alive.*
>
> —Howard Thurman

3. **Live in the Great Fullness of Life**, for when you are living in the Great Fullness of Life, you will relax into the flow of life where all is forgiven.

4. **Be Wholeness, Confidence, Joy, Fun, Graciousness, Generous, Abundance, Capable, Creative, Masterful, Thankful and Enthusiastic**, for when you are, you become the Song of Life and Life Sings through You.

This is the formula for Living a Meaningful Life. Go for it – for the entire world is waiting to hear your song.

**Being in the question – Take a moment to feel into:**

- ❖ What would it feel like to Be Love?
- ❖ What would it feel like to Shine My Brilliance?
- ❖ What would it feel like to Live in the Great Fullness of Life?
- ❖ What would it feel like to be Wholeness, Confidence, Joy, Fun, Graciousness, Masterful, Abundance, Capable, Creative, Thankful and Enthusiastic?

**Living Words:** Love, Fullness, Brilliance, Life, Wholeness, Confidence, Joy, Fun, Graciousness, Masterful, Abundance, Capable, Creative, Thankful and Enthusiastic.

*Don't say a thing.*
*Ecstasy, not words,*
*is the language spoken there.*

—**Rumi**

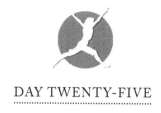

DAY TWENTY-FIVE

# Being Your Own Best Friend

What would it feel like to completely admire, respect, enjoy, trust and love yourself?

Today, spend some time in quiet reflection. Take a moment and journal about all the aspects you like about yourself such as: I am funny, honest, creative, generous, loving, thoughtful, intelligent, happy . . .

Spend time alone learning how to enjoy your own company. Have a **Private Party** walking in nature, diving into a new hobby or reading a great book. Feel into being alone and yet feeling complete, relaxed and happy.

Enjoy the quiet and freedom that comes with being your own best friend.

**Here is a list of the things I like about myself:**

I am: _____

_____

_____

_____

_____

_____

**Being in the question – Take a moment to feel into:**

- ❖ What does it feel like to admire myself?
- ❖ What does it feel like to truly respect myself?
- ❖ What does it feel like to fully love myself?
- ❖ What does it feel like to fully enjoy my own company?
- ❖ What does it feel like to be my own best friend?
- ❖ What does it feel like to feel whole?
- ❖ What does it feel like to feel safe?
- ❖ What does it feel like to know that I am enough?

**Living Words:** Friendship, Self-Respect, Trust, Happy, Inner Peace, Inner Joy and Freedom.

*Give yourself a kiss.*
*If you want to hold the beautiful one,*
*hold yourself to yourself.*

—**Rumi**

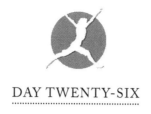

# Being Present

What if being present is a brilliant means for you to let go of worry?

What if all worry is about having your attention on the past or the future?

**Pause and Breathe:** A good way to stay present as you go through your day is to stop what you are doing, take a few slow, deep breaths, smile and check in with yourself. Feel into how you are feeling. Be present as you send Love to all that you are feeling, to the sadness along with the happiness.

**The Power of Silence/Stillness:** What if there is great power in silence and stillness? What if being in stillness brings on feelings of calm, completeness, centeredness, comfort, contentment and ease, while arousing the powers of creativity and manifestation?

**Finding Your Still Point:** Set aside 10 minutes and sit in a comfortable chair with your eyes closed. Take a few slow and deep breaths, and let your day go. Now, inhale slowly and deeply to the count of three, hold for the count of three, exhale to the count of three, and hold out for the count of three. Continue to breathe this way for 3–5 minutes. Your Still Point will be felt at the top of your inhale while you hold your breath for the three counts (be sure not to strain with this breathing). As you are breathing, put your attention on the center of your body two inches below your navel (this is the location of the Still Point in your body).

In time you may find that your life becomes filled with Blissful Calm, Inner Peace, feelings of Harmony, Happiness and Neutrality, and a soft, Joyful Smile bubbling up from your Inner Being!

The power of silence and stillness will become a part of your inner life, so practice the Still Point Breathing every day.

**Be Aware:** Take notice of your environment – the sounds, the sights, the taste, the touch, the smell.

**Revel in Beauty:** Be aware of all the beauty in everything – a mountain, a lake, a flower, a child, your friend, your body and the beauty of this magnificent creation we call life!

**The End of Multitasking:** Life can be much more enjoyable when you are focused on one thought or activity at a time. In his book, *The 7 Habits of Highly Effective People*, Stephen Covey states, "First things first." In other words, take all the action necessary to successfully accomplish the most important project, and then move on to the next.

Make a list of all that you aim to accomplish, in order of priority. When you successfully finish the first item on your list, cross it off, take a moment to celebrate your success, congratulate yourself on a job well done, then happily move on to your next project on the list.

There is a pure feeling of joy when you effectively accomplish something that is important to you.

**Being in Gratitude:** There is a luscious feeling of Joy and Being that will surround you when you are in full gratitude for all that is.

**Being in the question – Take a moment to feel into:**

- ❖ What would it feel like to be fully present?
- ❖ What would it feel like to completely enjoy the beauty that surrounds me?
- ❖ What would it feel like to give all of my attention to the task at hand?
- ❖ What would it feel like to complete all that I need to accomplish?

**Living Words:** Aware, Pause, Breathe, Still Point, Accomplish, Gratitude and Be.

*Look past your thoughts,*
*so you may drink the*
*pure nectar of This Moment.*

—Rumi

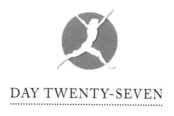

# Standing in Your Power

*Stepping Into Your Personal Power*

Standing in Your Power has nothing to do with control, dominance or power over someone. Standing in Your Power has everything to do with Standing in Your Courage, Your Patience, Your Wisdom, Your Certainty, Your Compassion, Your Joy, Your Clarity, Your Understanding, Your Depth, Your Abundance, Your Generosity, Your Love, Your Graciousness, Your Truth, Your Trust, Your Humility, Your Glory and Your God-Given Magnificence.

**Standing in Your Yes!** *Yes* gives you the power and glory of being in the Flow of Life. Use *Yes* often to bring more Beauty, Joy, Love and Grace into the world.

**Standing in Your No!** *No* gives you the power to stop the Flow of Life. Use *No* rarely, but whenever necessary, to set healthy boundaries.

**Flex Your Muscles with Grace and Kindness:** Trust yourself and feel into your power with Grace and Kindness. Step into Your Power with your inner confidence, and watch your Magnificence blossom.

**Being in the question – Take a moment to feel into:**

- ❖ What would it feel like to know my innate power?
- ❖ What would it feel like to know complete confidence?
- ❖ What would it feel like to know the power of Yes?
- ❖ What would it feel like to know the power of No?
- ❖ What would it feel like to stand in my Glory?

❖ What would it feel like to stand in my God-Given Magnificence?

**Living Words:** Power, Strength, Yes, No, Confidence, Generosity, Truth, Trust, Humility, Glory, Venerable and God-Given Magnificence.

*Come, seek, for search is the*
*foundation of fortune:*
*Every success depends upon*
*focusing the heart.*

**—Rumi**

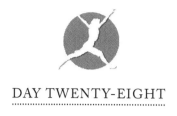

## DAY TWENTY-EIGHT

# Stand-Up Comedian

Everyone likes to laugh. And we all know that "Laughter is the best medicine." A good laugh stimulates the production of "Joy Juices" in your body such as endorphins, dopamine, oxytocin and serotonin.

So become an Ellen Degeneres, a Jerry Seinfeld and a Jimmy Fallon, by telling funny stories and jokes.

Bring a new joke to work each week and get your coworkers rolling on the floor.

You will find thousands of good jokes online.

Even better, search for "funny videos," and every week send the funniest video to your Joy Club and your Facebook friends.

**Here are some fun one-liners:**

- ❖ What do alligators drink before a race? Gator-Ade.
- ❖ What do you call an alligator that sneaks up and bites you from behind? A tail-gater.
- ❖ What do yuppie alligators like to drink? Jaw-va.
- ❖ What do you call an alligator that causes trouble? An Insti-gator.
- ❖ Why don't cats like online shopping? They prefer a cat-alogue.
- ❖ There were 10 cats in a boat and one jumped out. How many were left? None, because they were copycats!
- ❖ What is smarter than a talking cat? A spelling bee!
- ❖ Why was the cat sitting on the computer? To keep an eye on the mouse!

Okay, you may want to save these jokes for your five-year-old friends.

*The secret of staying young is to live honestly, eat slowly, and lie about your age.*

—Lucille Ball

*Everything you see here I owe to spaghetti.*

—Sophia Loren

**So laugh!** Choose to spend time with friends who make you laugh and with friends who laugh at your jokes. Collect a joke every week to Tweet, post on your Facebook page and share with everyone who could use a good laugh—(we all could use a good laugh).

**Being in the question – Take a moment to feel into:**

❖ What would it feel like to laugh so hard that tears run down your face?

❖ What would it feel like to laugh so hard that you and your friends are rolling on the floor?

❖ What would it feel like to know that you are a fun and funny person?

**Living Words:** Fun, Laugh, Make Them Laugh and Make Them Cry.

*What is this precious love and laughter
budding in our hearts?*

*It is the sound of a soul waking up!*

*Even after all this time, the sun never
says to the earth, "You owe me."*

*Look what happens with a love like that,
It lights up the whole sky.*

—Rumi

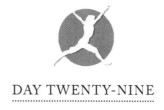

# Time to Reflect and to Integrate

**W**OW: Here you are on day 29!

You have come a long way: you are experiencing more smiles, more love, more gratitude, more grace, more adventure, more power, more laughs and more inner peace.

Today will be wholly devoted to reflecting on where you were 29 days ago, in contrast to where you are now. It will be a time for you to relax into the joyful feelings for all that you have accomplished, and to look for ways to integrate the growth and knowledge that you have gained over the past 29 days, into your daily life.

This is your time to look back and reflect upon all the areas in which you have grown and how your life now expresses more Joy, Abundance and Freedom. Seek to bring an essence of all that you have gained into every thought, every word and every action from this day forward.

Here is how my life has expanded into new Joys, Abundance and Freedom:

## Day 1 – Self-Love
**I am**

_____

_____

_____

## Day 2 – Shake Your Body
I am

_____

_____

_____

## Day 3 – Good Vibrations
I am

_____

_____

_____

## Day 4 – Your Life Story
I am

_____

_____

_____

## Day 5 – Passion
I am

_____

_____

_____

# Day 6 – Living Words

I am

_____

_____

_____

_____

# Day 7 – Friendship – Feeling Fully Supported

I am

_____

_____

_____

_____

# Day 8 – Putting Yourself First –
# Time For You To Shine!

I am

_____

_____

_____

_____

## Day 9 – Love for No Reason – Joy for No Reason

I am

_____

_____

_____

## Day 10 – Living Healthy – Healthy Living

I am

_____

_____

_____

## Day 11 – Anger, Rage, Hate, Guilt, Shame, Sadness

I am

_____

_____

_____

## Day 12 – Forgiveness – Letting Go

I am

_____

_____

_____

## Day 13 – Making Friends with God

I am

_____

_____

_____

## Day 14 – Meditation

I am

_____

_____

_____

## Day 15 – Beauty

I am

_____

_____

_____

## Day 16 – Adventure

I am

_____

_____

_____

# Day 17 – Abundance
### I am

_____

_____

_____

# Day 18 – Fun
### I am

_____

_____

_____

# Day 19 – Romance
### I am

_____

_____

_____

# Day 20 – Take The Day Off
### I am

_____

_____

_____

# Day 23 – Create
I am

_____

_____

_____


# Day 24 – Living a Meaningful Life
I am

_____

_____

_____


# Day 25 – Being Your Own Best Friend
I am

_____

_____

_____


# Day 26 – Being Present
I am

_____

_____

_____

## Day 27 – Standing in Your Power

### I am

_____

_____

_____

## Day 28 – Stand-Up Comedian

### I am

_____

_____

_____

## Day 29 – A Time to Reflect and To Integrate

### I am

_____

_____

_____

## Day 30 – Thrive: You Made It!

### I am

_____

_____

_____

*In every moment, in every event of your life,*
*the Beloved is whispering to you exactly*
*what you need to hear and know.*
*Who can ever explain this miracle?*
*It simply is. Listen and you will discover*
*it every passing moment.*
*Listen, and your whole life will become*
*a conversation in thought and act between*
*you and Him,*
*directly, wordlessly, now and always.*

—Rumi

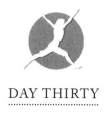

# Thrive: You Made It!

*In Love – At Joy*
*Celebrating Your Love and Joy – Being Thankful*

WOW! You made it through 30 days of playing, crying, seeking, dancing, eating, breathing, Being, Loving and laughing. There is no need to look back, only to be present to the new Love and Joy in your life. Take time this week to celebrate your new life, to be proud of yourself, and to give thanks for all that you have gained. Call up your family and closest friends and invite them to have a good time in your honor at your Joy Party.

Take a full week to bathe in your newly found delight of *Being: Being Love, Being Joy, Being Happy and Being Healthy.*

Relax into life, revel in who you are, experience your Joy and be Thankful and Content.

**Empowering My Life With Joy:** Here are six new ways that Joy will be a part of my life from this day forward:

1. _____

   _____

2. _____

   _____

3. _____

_____

4. _____

_____

5. _____

_____

6. _____

_____

**Taking Your Life to a Higher Level:** Life is a magnificent journey, and there is always more to learn, more growing to do, and greater levels of Love and Joy to experience. So go for it!

Take a few weeks off, and bask in your new life. Then take your life to a higher level of Love and Joy by gathering a group of close friends and jumping into this 30-day adventure *For The Love Of Joy* one more time! You will gain new Love, more Joy, brighter Light and a fuller Life.

**Develop and Live a Daily Routine** that brings you more Love, Joy and better Health. Make this Daily Routine fun and within your capabilities. For ideas, check out the Daily Routine on the next page.

**Selfie:** Today, take a picture of yourself and post it on page viii in this book, below the photo you took on the first day of this adventure into greater Joy. Is your smile more joyful; do your eyes shine brighter; do you look more confident, calm and complete?

> **Remember, as long as you are moving closer to Joy and bringing more Love and Beauty into your Life, you are as good as Gold!**

**Being in the question – Take a moment to feel into:**

- ❖ What would it feel like to be content in Life?
- ❖ What would it feel like to be Happy, Joyous and Loving?
- ❖ What would it feel like to take my life to an even higher level?
- ❖ What would it feel like to fully like myself?
- ❖ What would it feel like to be truly Thankful for who I Am?
- ❖ What would it feel like to be fully Proud of myself for all that I have accomplished over these 30 days?

**Living Words:** Celebrate, Joy, Love, Thankful, Complete, Confident, Brilliant, Magnificent and Alive!

*I am in Love with Love*
*and Love is in Love with me.*
*My body is in Love with the soul*
*and the soul is in Love with my body.*
*I opened my arms to Love*
*and Love embraced me like a lover.*

—Rumi

# Create Your Own Daily Routine

The following is a recommended daily routine designed to bring more Health, Fun and Joy into your life. Please feel free to add your special touch to your daily routine – include whatever will bring a Smile to your face and Joy to your Heart!

**Remember:** Early to bed (by 10:00 p.m., or 11:00 p.m. at the latest) and early to rise (7:00 a.m.).

## Morning

**Prayer before rising:** Recite your own personal prayer, or you can say: "This is the day that the Lord has made, I will rejoice and be happy therein. Dear God, what Love, Joy, Beauty and Peace can I bring into the world today?"

**Start Your Day With Joy, Gratitude and Love!** With your eyes closed, when your first wake up, feel into a few moments of pure Gratitude, being thankful as you count your many blessings. Next, envision all of the Joys that you would like to experience over the next 24 hours. Smile as you feel in your heart and your body the joyfulness of all the Yums and Wows that you would like to experience today.

- ❖ Wake up like a lion doing a Happy Dance.
- ❖ Journal your intentions for the day.
- ❖ Shower with I Love Yous.
- ❖ Full-Body Massage with essential oils (lavender, sweet orange, rose or peppermint).
- ❖ Exercise: Yoga, Qigong or a morning walk.
- ❖ Morning Meditation.

- ❖ Healthy breakfast: Offer a prayer of Gratitude before and after eating, enjoying each bite.
- ❖ Smile as you go through your day.

# Afternoon

**A Moment Of Joy – Join The Joy Revolution:** At 12-noon every day, spend a few minutes in Joy, Love and Gratitude. This is a fun way to raise feelings of Joy in yourself, while simultaneously raising the level of Joy in the world. Spend a few minutes in silent Joy at noon each day, feeling into all that you are grateful for, and all that you Love. Send Love and Healing to a friend who is hurting or to a nation whose citizens are hurting, such as the people living in the Middle East. If you are out to lunch with friends, ask them to talk about the Joys and Loves in their lives. Make a list of the new Joys that you can bring into your life and into the lives of others.

- ❖ Healthy lunch: Say a prayer of Gratitude before and after eating, and savor each bite.
- ❖ Fun and laughter: Bring some fun and laughter into your day and into the day of those in your life.
- ❖ Exercise: Twenty minutes or more.
- ❖ Afternoon Meditation.

# Evening

- ❖ Healthy dinner: Say a prayer of appreciation before and after eating, while enjoying each bite.
- ❖ Family time: Enjoy learning and playing together; plan your next week, month, year, and your family vacation to Italy.
- ❖ Quiet time (all electronics turned off): Relax while reading, meditating, reflecting, journaling and laughing.
- ❖ Bedtime: Journal your intentions for the next day, offer a prayer of Gratitude and sail into happy thoughts as you swim into sleep.

# My Morning Routine:

_____

_____

_____

_____

_____

_____

_____

_____

_____

_____

_____

_____

_____

_____

_____

# My Afternoon Routine:

_____

_____

_____

_____

_____

_____

_____

_____

_____

_____

_____

_____

_____

_____

_____

# My Evening Routine:

_____

_____

_____

_____

_____

_____

_____

_____

_____

_____

_____

_____

_____

_____

# Weekly Routine

*Improving Your Life One Week at a Time*

Once a week, devote one to two hours (perhaps every Sunday morning), to making your life better. Look for projects that are waiting for your loving attention, such as: Organizing your closet, purse/wallet, office, finances—(saving an extra hundred bucks, giving an extra twenty dollars to someone in need); writing that letter that you have been putting off; or taking the necessary steps to repair a strained relationship. Feel how good you feel when each week of your life becomes more enjoyable as you take care of the "little things" that are calling for your attention.

# Joyful Resources – For Joyful Living

The Following resources are extremely valuable tools that will help increase Joy in all areas of your life, including health, wealth, wisdom and inner peace.

## Energy Healers:

The following are highly skilled energy healers:

**Jo Dunning:** www.JoDunning.com – *Discovering The Love You Are.* Jo has a soft yet powerful ability to help you remove emotional blocks so that you can propel your life forward with love and joy.

**Rikka Zimmerman**: www.Rikka Zimmerman.com – *Adventures In Oneness: Awaken To A New World.* Rikka is a remarkable healer on an emotional and physical level. She has helped thousands of people to become abundant in health and wealth by helping them raise their vibrations.

**Matt Kahn:** www.TrueDivineNature.com – *The Love Revolution.* Matt offers you deep wisdom and easy to follow techniques to bring about more joy in your life.

**Panache Desai:** www.PanacheDesai.com – *Stepping Out Of Fear And Limitations: Experiencing Your Deepest Connection and True Potential.* Panache conveys a very special energy that will assist in lifting you to higher levels of joy and healing.

**Marie Manuchehri:** www.EnergyIntuitive.com – *Intuitive Self-Healing: Achieve Balance and Wellness Through the Body's Energy Centers.* Marie has a put together a series of CDs that will give you great insights into how to heal yourself.

## Healing Music:

The following musicians have a worldwide reputation for composing and playing inspiring music, which raises the vibration in human physiology, enabling one to be happier, healthier and more peaceful.

**Barry Goldstein:** www.BarryGoldsteinMusic.com. Barry has a very special talent for infusing the Universal Power of Love into his music.

**Jim Oliver:** www.JimOliverMusic.com. Jim brings together healing sound and color to uplift one's body and soul.

**Jonathan Goldman**: www.HealingSounds.com. Jonathan has a large selection of courses and music downloads that will open you to higher levels of Joy and Healing.

**Steve Halpern:** www.SteveHalpern.com. Steve's special music will offer you vibrations that are relaxing, healing, meditative and will help to bring on restful sleep.

## Abundance:

*Financial Peace University* by Dave Ramsey, **www.DaveRamsey. com**. Dave Ramsey offers you a complete financial plan for getting your finances in order, from getting out of debt to building a large money reserve that will help you feel at peace with your finances.

*Think and Grow Rich* by Napoleon Hill, **www.Naphill.org**. This book will help direct your thinking and actions, inspiring you to live a more financially abundant life.

*Yes to Success!* By Debra Poneman, **www.YesToSuccess.com**. Debra has been helping people live more successful and happier lives for over 30 years.

## Essential Oils:

Caution: Essential Oils can be very powerful. It is best to dilute them in a base oil such as grape seed oil or olive oil before applying the oil to your skin. To learn more, please consult with a certified Aromatherapist in your area.

**Young Living**, www.YoungLiving.com. Young Living offers very high quality oils with many great oil blends including: Joy, Abundance, Acceptance, Harmony, Forgiveness and Fun.

**Aromatics International**, www.Aromatics.com. Aromatics International has a nice selection of high quality, all organic oils.

## Qi Gong:

*Awakening The Soul.* This is a powerful yet easy ten-minute sitting Qi Gong exercise where you follow the master's moves.

   You will find it on You Tube at: **www.youtube.com/ watch?v=o8LxAS-eJdg**. Or you may Google: *Awakening The Soul.*

## Helpful Reads:

*The Passion Test*, created by Chris Attwood and Janet Bray Attwood, **www.ThePassionTest.com**, will provide you with clear, simple and effective techniques to help you recognize your core passions. This will assist you in creating a happy, meaningful and purpose-filled life. Once you identify and live your passions, watch out – life will get very exciting.

*Happy for No Reason: 7 Steps to Being Happy from the Inside Out*, by Marci Shimoff offers you a breakthrough approach to being happy. This book incorporates the latest findings in positive psychology, powerful tools and techniques, moving real-life stories and a 7-step program that will raise your "happiness set-point."

*Conversations With God*, by Neale Donald Walsch, **www.CWG.org**, is a best selling book, with over seven million copies sold. This book is easy to read and offers you great insights to some of life's most profound questions such as the nature of God, love, faith, life, death, good and your life's purpose.

*Calling In The One*, by Katherine Woodward Thomas, wwwKatherineWoodwardThomas.com.

*The Soulmate Secret: Three Keys To Manifesting True Love*, by Arielle Ford, www.ArielleFord.com.

*Whatever Arises, Love That: A Love Revolution That Begins With You*, by Matt Kahn, **www.TrueDivineNature.com**. Matt Kahn is an empathic healer who offers you meaningful insights that will add charm to your life. In his new book, he richly explores ways to help you bring your highest self forward in all that life brings you.

*The Bible:* What if being in the word of God will bring you closer to Him?

## Meditation:

Transcendental Meditation. **www.TM.org.**

Stillness. **www.TheStillnessProject.com**

## Healthy Living – Living Healthy

## Juicing:

Juicing organic fresh fruits and vegetables is a great way to improve your health and energy. All you need is a juicer or a blender ($50-$500), fresh fruits and vegetables ($2-$10), and time (Free). Have fun making up your own blends or check out the Internet for the more traditional recipes.

Two good starter juicing books are: *Juicing for Health: How to use natural juices to boost energy, immunity, and wellbeing*, by Caroline Wheater and *101 Juice Recipes*, by Joe Cross.

## Sprouting:

**Sprout People,** www.SproutPeople.org, offers you a Beginner's Starter Kit ($39.93) that contains everything you need in order to grow great sprouts at home, including the Easy Sprout container and seeds. Sprouts are fun and easy to grow and they are also a living food full of minerals, vitamins, Omega 3s, Omega 6s and protein. There are a full variety of sprouting seeds to choose from, such as lentil, mung bean, radish, alfalfa, broccoli and clover. Each seed has a different taste and nutritional composition.

## Clean Water:

**Filtered Water Pitchers** can be found online. It is best to purchase one that reduces chlorine, flouride and heavy metals from your tap water.

## Organic Foods can be found at any health food store.

## Vitamins and Supplements:

**Youngevity, www.Youngevity.com**, offers you a full range of the highest quality vitamins, minerals, and Omega 3 oils.

## Healthy Living Websites:

**Mind Body Green**, www.MindBodyGreen.com, gives you useful information on most every topic, to guide you to a healthier life.

**Gaia**, www.Gaia.com, ($10 a month membership), has a full array of tips for healthy living, from easy yoga at home, to healthy eating, to living your life in balance.

## Free Daily Webinars Bringing You Inspirational Speakers and Healers:

*The You Wealth Revolution* hosted by Darius Barazandeh, www.YouWealthRevolution.com

*From Heartache To Joy* hosted by Eram Saeed, www.FromHeartacheToJoy.com

*Healing With The Masters* hosted by Jennifer McLean, www.HealingWithThe Masters.com

*Beyond The Ordinary Show* hosted by John Burgos, www.BeyondTheOrdinaryShow.com

*Energized Living Today* hosted by Cindy Kubica, **www.EnergizedLivingToday.com**

# A Global Moment of Joy!

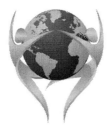

## Helping to Create a More Joyful and Peaceful World

### *One Billion People In Joy*

At 12-noon everyday, spend some time in Joy, Love and Gratitude. This is a fun way to raise feelings of Joy in yourself, while also raising the level of Joy in the world. Spend a few minutes in Joy at noon each day, feeling into all that you are grateful for, or all that you Love. You may also send *Love* to a friend who is hurting or to a nation whose citizens are hurting, such as the people living in the Middle East, to help create a more peaceful world. For anywhere there is more Love, there is more Joy and Peace.

**Joy in Motion – Taking Action:** Think of ways to bring more Joy into your life and into the life of someone else, then go and make it happen. Every day, look for ways that you can bring one new Joy into your life and into the life of another. If you are out to lunch with friends, ask them to talk about the Joys and Loves in their lives, and how they feel that they can bring more Joy into their lives and into the lives of others. Spread the Joy!

**Be a Joy Ambassador:** Share *A Global Moment of Joy* with your friends and family and with everyone in your social media realm, and encourage them to join in on the fun.

The goal of a Joy Ambassador is to help raise the level of Joy in all life on earth and by being one of the millions of people in each time zone around the world engaging in a *Global Moment of Joy*. Think of the powerful energy that forms when millions of people come together every day in Joy, Love and Gratitude.

## The Power of Social Media – Spreading the Joy to One Billion People Around the World

Let's say you invite 100 of your friends to be Joy Ambassadors = 100.

...They invite 100 of their friends = 10,000

...Then the 10,000 invite 100 of their friends = 1,000,000

...Then the 1,000,000 invite 100 of their friends = 100,000,000

...And then the 100,000,000 invite 10 of their friends = **One Billion People bringing Joy, Love and Gratitude into the World!!!**

## So help spread the word and be a part of creating a more Peaceful and Joyful World.

Learn more at: **www.GlobalMomentOfJoy.com**